Communication Sciences
# Student Survival Guide

This guide is dedicated to students in communication sciences and disorders programs who are trying to figure out what to do to survive.

This guide is also dedicated to all student mentors, especially Francine Emmons, CCC-SLP, who generously mentored me from high school through graduate school.

*Marie Patton*

# Communication Sciences
# Student Survival Guide

## National Student Speech Language Hearing Association

Edited by Marie A. Patton

**THOMSON**

**DELMAR LEARNING**    Australia   Canada   Mexico   Singapore   Spain   United Kingdom   United States

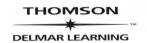

# Communication Sciences Student Survival Guide

Edited by Marie A. Patton

**Vice President Health Care Business Unit:**
William Brottmiller

**Editorial Director:**
Cathy L. Esperti

**Acquisitions Editor:**
Kalen Conerly

**Marketing Director:**
Jennifer McAvey

**Developmental Editor:**
Juliet Byington

**Marketing Coordinator:**
Chris Manion

**Production Editor:**
James Zayicek

**Library of Congress Cataloging-in-Publication Data**

Communication sciences student survival guide / National Student Speech Language Hearing Association ; edited by Marie A. Patton.
    p. cm.
    Includes bibliographical references and index.
    ISBN 1-4018-8256-0
    1. Audiology--Vocational guidance. 2. Speech therapy--Vocational guidance. 3. Communicative disorders--Study and teaching. I. Title: Student survival guide. II. Patton, Marie A. III. National Student Speech Language Hearing Association (U.S.)

RC428.5.C65 2004
616.85'5023--dc22

                                                        2004056010

## NOTICE TO THE READER

# Contents

# Preface

*Communication Sciences Student Survival Guide* is a must-have resource for individuals considering a future in the disciplines of audiology, speech-language pathology, or speech-language-hearing sciences. This guide is a relevant and useful tool for individuals who are at any point along the path toward a career in communication sciences and disorders (CSD). By providing practical advice from students and professionals in CSD, users learn everything from the differences in CSD degrees, to how to choose and get into the right educational program, to how to be successful as an undergraduate, graduate student, and professional. In addition, mentors of students in CSD will find this to be a valuable resource for its many tips and tricks, including contact information for a wide range of CSD programs, listing of pertinent Web sites, and suggested readings. This comprehensive guide will be an invaluable companion for anyone thinking about, or pursuing, a successful career in these exciting professions.

## REASON FOR THIS GUIDE

This project started as a booklet that the National Student Speech Language Hearing Association's (NSSLHA's) Executive Council sought to create to meet the needs of NSSLHA's members. When the editor was a Regional Councilor during her junior year of college, she read a proposed table of contents and began brainstorming other topics that would be useful and thought-provoking. Months later, she read the draft of the document, which included approximately ten pages of advice for undergraduates and master's students. It was a great start, but it needed more advice and content areas, so material was added and students from various universities were invited to review the document and offer suggestions. An active dialogue was started and ultimately, other content areas, such as advice for doctoral students, why it is important to take both audiology and SLP courses, clinical fellowships, and the job outlook were added. The NSSLHA Executive Council and Director of Operations, Dawn Dickerson, also provided invaluable feedback and contributions to the growing document. Approximately three years after Marie Patton's initial encounter, this comprehensive, practical guide has been completed with the assistance of over 150 students and professionals.

# HOW THIS TEXT IS ORGANIZED

*Communication Sciences Student Survival Guide* is broken out into four sections: introductory and background information on communication sciences, information for specific areas and levels of study, career path guidance and professional issues, and appendices.

The beginning chapters cover basic information, such as what an audiologist is, what a speech-language pathologist does, and what the job market looks like for individuals with different CSD degrees. There is also information on financing a CSD education, with great tips on finding and applying for scholarships, grants, and loans.

The next chapters provide advice specific to individuals at different points in their CSD education, such as "Chapter 6, Advice for High School Students," "Chapter 7, Advice for Freshman Year," and continues through advice for graduate and doctoral level students in different degree programs. The advice chapters can be used as checklists of important things to do or consider during each year of one's education. While some advice is appropriate for more than one group of students and is shared in multiple chapters, each chapter also provides tips and strategies that are unique to its particular audience.

The final chapters provide engaging interviews with professionals working in a wide range of settings. These interviews provide a glimpse into the day-to-day experiences of audiologists, speech-language pathologists, and speech-language-hearing scientists, and are a great way to learn more about areas of specialization. There are also chapters with specific advice on seeking a job (e.g., writing a resumé and interviewing) and how to be involved with national organizations as a professional (e.g., American Speech-Language-Hearing Association).

The appendices are some of the most exciting features in the book. The most robust appendix, Appendix B, Undergraduate and Graduate Programs in CSD, provides a state-by-state listing of colleges and universities offering degree programs in CSD. Contact information for each school is provided, and a key indicates what degrees the school offers (i.e., undergraduate, Au.D., master's SLP), as well as any additional significant information about that school (bilingual or minority focus, or distance learning program). This appendix is an excellent starting point for anyone investigating potential programs. The other appendices offer a variety of useful tools as well. For example, Appendix A lists materials that can assist individuals in being organized. Appendix C provides a list of suggested readings related to CSD. Appendix F provides a list of key acronyms and phrases that individuals encounter in the field (e.g., ASHA, IEP, CF, and Au.D.); however, these acronyms do not include diagnoses and treatments because that is beyond the scope of this guide.

Although this guide discusses the CSD degree at the very beginning and follows the different career paths through to the many different professional possibilities that exist, individuals at any point in their academic career can jump into the text and get invaluable advice.

# HOW TO USE THIS GUIDE

The unique advantage of this book is that it does not have to be read from front to back. It is designed for individuals to access information as needed throughout their academic journey. For example, an individual who is just considering a career in CSD might begin with the introduction and job outlook chapters. These chapters explain the professions of audiology and speech-language pathology and how promising the job outlooks are. Depending upon an individual's place in life (e.g., college student, post-bachelor's, nurse, engineer), the reader can look in the table of contents for the advice chapter that best applies.

Once an individual reads the chapter, or chapters, that most directly applies to him or her, subsequent advice chapters can be read to prepare for the next academic step (e.g., sophomores can read the junior, senior, and master's/doctoral chapters). Reading these chapters will assist a student in knowing what to expect in his or her academic future.

Most individuals in CSD would benefit from reading the chapters on scholarships and financial support, transitioning from undergraduate to graduate coursework, writing for the clinical practicum, research basics, specialty interests, other career options in CSD, resumé and interview preparation, and advice for choosing a clinical fellowship. The resumé and interview preparation chapter also includes advice on applying for a faculty or clinical supervisor position in CSD.

A useful feature of this guide is the worksheets included in some chapters. For example, in the chapter on advice for freshmen, readers can fill out the contact information worksheet, which includes spaces for professors, mentors, and names of student and professional organizations. In the chapter on advice for seniors, the worksheet will assist in keeping track of graduate application deadlines and contact information. These tools can be photocopied for personal use and are intended to help organize important information.

Mentors, including faculty members, NSSLHA leaders, high school guidance counselors, and any individual who might want to be a mentor, would benefit from reading this guide. Mentors and guidance counselors can share the ideas that would be helpful to students considering and/or studying CSD, and design their mentoring or guidance programs to reflect this advice.

Of course, reading the entire book will help one get the most complete picture of the academic requirements and the profession as a whole, but this guide can be tailored to met any individual's needs.

# AVENUE FOR FEEDBACK

Anyone who has questions, suggestions, or comments about the guide can contact the NSSLHA National Office at nsslha@asha.org. NSSLHA welcomes students who have more advice and experiences to share for the guide. NSSLHA and the editor hope the *Communication Sciences Student Survival Guide* provides you with support, advice, and encouragement, and wish you the best of luck in your academic programs and your professional career.

## ABOUT THE EDITOR, MARIE A. PATTON, BHS

Currently, Marie Patton is a master's student in speech-language pathology at the University of Wisconsin-Madison. She completed her Bachelor's of Health Sciences in Communication Disorders at the University of Kentucky. She not only has experience as a student in CSD, but experience with student and professional organizations at the local, state, and national levels.

Marie knew she wanted to be a speech-language pathologist during high school when she read about the profession at a local public library and then observed a speech-language pathologist (Francine Emmons). As a freshman in college, she joined the University of Kentucky's NSSLHA chapter, and continued her membership until graduation. During her sophomore year, Marie was elected Regional Councilor for the NSSLHA Executive Council and she volunteered at the Kentucky Speech-Language-Hearing Association's office in Lexington, KY. During her junior year, Marie was elected President of NSSLHA. As part of this position, she was a voting member on the ASHA Legislative Council. During the spring of her junior year, she started working on this guide and continued to add to the text each semester, as she gained more advice from peers and had more experiences. During her senior year, Marie was editor of the local NSSLHA chapter's newsletter.

As a graduate student at the University of Wisconsin-Madison, Marie has been a member of the local NSSLHA chapter and editor of the newsletter. She has spoken at four state conventions and two teleseminars on topics related to leadership and advice for students. Most recently, Marie has attended five state conventions and three ASHA conventions. She is also a project assistant and has an interest in Augmentative and Alternative Communication. After graduation, Marie plans to work for a few years before returning to school for a Ph.D.

# Contributors

Marie A. Patton, BHS
*Communication Sciences Student Survival Guide* Editor and Coordinator
NSSLHA President, 2002–2003; NSSLHA Regional Councilor, 2001–2003; ASHA Legislative Councilor, 2002–2003
Graduate student in speech-language pathology at the University of Wisconsin-Madison

Nichole Castle
Graduate student in speech-language pathology at Eastern Washington University

Michelle Cox, MA, CCC-SLP
Doctorate of Philosophy candidate in Composition Studies at the University of New Hampshire

Lee Cruz
Assistant Director of Placement Services in Counseling and Career Services at Saint Xavier University

Vicki Deal-Williams, MA, CCC-SLP
ASHA Chief Staff Officer for Multicultural Affairs

Dawn D. Dickerson, MPA
NSSLHA Director of Operations

Erica Dmuchoski, BS
NSSLHA Regional Councilor, 2001–2003; ASHA Council on Clinical Certification, 2002
Au.D. candidate at Central Michigan University

Kelly Farquharson
NSSLHA Regional Councilor, 2003–2005
Graduate student in speech-language pathology at Pennsylvania State University

Larissa Fedak, BS
NSSLHA Regional Councilor, 2002–2004
Graduate student in special education at New Jersey City University

Jeremy Federman, BS
NSSLHA Regional Councilor, Region III, 2003–2005
Graduate student in hearing sciences at Vanderbilt University

Cynthia Gannett, Ph.D.
Director of Writing Across the Curriculum at Loyola College

Jeanette Glenn, BS
Graduate student in audiology at the University of Wisconsin-Madison

Sharon Goodson, MS, CCC-A
NSSLHA President, 2000–2002; NSSLHA Regional Councilor, Region X, 2000–2002; ASHA Legislative Councilor, 2001–2002
Graduated from San Francisco State University

Caryn Neuvrith, BS
NSSLHA President, 2003–2004; ASHA Legislative Councilor, 2003–2004
Sc.D. candidate in audiology at Seton Hall University

Kristi L. Pennypacker, BS
Graduate student in speech-language
pathology at Bloomsburg University

Amy Solomon Plante, MEd, CCC-SLP
Clinical Assistant Professor at the University
of New Hampshire

Jeremy Saylor
Undergraduate in speech-language pathology
at the University of Kentucky

Jeanne O'Sullivan, MEd, CCC-SLP
Clinical Assistant Professor at the University
of New Hampshire

Sheri Tracy
Graduate student in speech-language
pathology at the University of Wisconsin-
Madison

Sherri Webster, BA
Graduate student in speech-language
pathology at Western Washington
University

# Acknowledgments

I would like to thank every student and professional who has assisted with this book. I would especially like to thank Dawn Dickerson, NSSLHA Director of Operations, and Larissa Fedak, NSSLHA Regional Councilor, who spent many long days and nights assisting me in completing various drafts of this guide. I would like to thank Mary Fleming, who assisted me in writing the proposal to Delmar Learning for this book.

*—Marie Patton*

## NSSLHA EXECUTIVE COUNCIL

Thank you to each of the NSSLHA Executive Council members who were involved with the creation of this guide:

Lauren Bland, Multicultural Consultant, 2000–2006

Anthony Caruso, Editor, 1998–2005

Erica Dmuchoski, Regional Councilor, Region I, 2001–2003

Diana Elizabeth Diaz, Regional Councilor, Region IX, 2001–2003

Larissa Fedak, Regional Councilor, Region II, 2002–2004

Jeremy Federman, Regional Councilor, Region III, 2003–2005

Lynn Flahive, Executive Director, 1999–2004

Tonya Foster, Regional Councilor, Region VII, 2002–2004

Amber Gaines, Vice President, Region V, 1999–2001

Nakiesha Giorgis, Vice-President, Region V, 2000–2002

Elyse Greenebaum, Regional Councilor, Region II, 2001–2003

Lindy Michelle Griffith, Regional Councilor, Region VIII, 1999–2001

Katherine Ann Haddix, Regional Councilor, Region IV, 2001–2003

Micah Johnson, Regional Councilor, Region IX, 1999–2001

Judi Keller, Convention Consultant, 2000–2006

Jacquie Kurland, Vice-President, Region II, 1999–2001

Rachel Mikles, President, Region VI, 1999–2002

Caryn Neuvirth, President, Region V, 2002–2005

Wesley Nicholson, Vice-President, Region X, 2002–2004

Jean Novak, Consultant at Large, 1998–2004

Rachel Parlier, Regional Councilor, Region VII, 2000–2002

Marie A. Patton, President, Regional Councilor, Region III, 2001–2004

Shannon Pfaff, Regional Councilor, Region X, 1999–2001

Jennifer Rayburn, Regional Councilor, Region III, 1998–2001

Keenya Rudd, Regional Councilor, Region VIII, 2002–2004

Tina Scaccia, Regional Councilor, Region II, 2000–2002

Whitney Schneider, Regional Councilor, Region VI, 2003–2005

Tricia Simpkins, Regional Councilor, Region VIII, 2000–2002

Scott Smith, Vice President, Region IV, 1999–2001

Bobbie Kay Smithson, Vice-President, Regional
Councilor, Region IX, 2003–2005

Sharon Sprugasci Goodson, President, Region X,
2000–2003

Beverly Straub, Regional Councilor, Region I,
1999–2001

Andrew D. Towers, Vice-President, Regional
Councilor, Region VI, 2001–2003

Nicole Villanueva, President, Region IV,
2003–2006

Michelle Williams, Regional Councilor, Region VII,
1999–2001

## STUDENTS

NSSLHA expresses a very special thank you to the following students and
recent graduates who have assisted in the completion of this guide.

Laura Anderson, University of Wisconsin-
Madison

Cynthia Andrews, California State University-
Fullerton

Jamie Lynn Azcona, Hofstra University

Patti Bailey, Towson State University

Mandi Barnes, University of Kentucky

Kelly Beck

Jennifer Benedik, University of Vermont

Deanene Berry

Jennifer Bohannan, Louisiana Tech University

Mary Brooks, Western Virginia University

Kristina Brzyski

Barbara Cardeso, Florida International University

Myesha Carter, University of the District of
Columbia

Nichole D. Castle, Eastern Washington University

Amanda J. Cerka, Northwestern University

Gwen Hallman Christensen, California University
of Pennsylvania

Melissa Coverston, Florida State University

Jessamyn Crade, University of Wisconsin-
Madison

Rena Cureton, Governor's State University

Nasim Dehghani, University of Utah

Sarah Dick, Thiel College

Mary Fleming, St. Xavier University

Amy Francek, Temple University

Renee R. Graff, Nova Southeastern University

Sheila L. Graham, CUNY-Hunter College

Jennifer Bohannan Green, Louisiana Tech
University

Lauren Gutstein, Boston University

Lisa Harrison, University of New Hampshire

Darla Hagge, California State University-Fullerton

Michelle Hall, University of Kentucky

Andrea Hoover, Wichita State University

Kimberly Ann Kiss, University of Wisconsin-
Madison

Joy Kling, CUNY-Queens College

Lindsay Knobelauch, University of Virginia-
Charlottesville

Candace Kukino, University of Washington

Ingrid Larson, University of Kentucky

Jennifer Lehnen, Old Dominion University

Adria B. Leno, University of Wisconsin-Madison

Claire Lombardo

Liza Martiniello, Ithaca College

Rachel Mattingly, Kent State University

Kimberly M. Meigh, University of Pittsburgh

Scott Miller, San Diego State University

Monique Mills, Ohio State University

Shari Moore, University of Arizona

Kyu Eun Na

Marnel N. Niles

Janice O'Brien

Alesia Okeke, Eastern Michigan University

Maureen S. Orawiec, Indiana University-
Bloomington

Beverly A. Page, Valdosta State University

Heather M. Powers, University of Tennessee-
Knoxville

Lindsay Quinn, Northern Arizona University

Lesley Raisor, University of Cincinnati

Kristin B. Reisch, SUNY College at Fredonia

Anastasia G. Reiter, University of Wisconsin-
Madison

Willow Sauermilch, University of Houston

Ursulla Schiller, Northern Illinois University

Whitney Settles, University of Kentucky

Kanika So, University of Wisconsin-Madison

Emily Spurk, Edinboro University

Sally Stevens, University of Arizona

Sarah Jane Stout, Utah State University

Jill Stubblefield, James Madison University
Katherine Sumner, Butler University
Megan Amalia Szmajda, Louisiana State
University
Barbara Tirado, CUNY-Queens College

Ted Trenkamp, Northern Illinois University
Kathryn L. Ward, Rockhurst University
Nicole Wiessner, California State University
Northridge
Niki Woodward, University of Utah

## PROFESSIONALS

NSSLHA expresses appreciation to the following researchers, clinicians, professors, and staff who have assisted in the completion of this guide.

Paul J. Abbas, Ph.D., University of Iowa
Kelly Appler, ASHA Associate Director of
Credentialing
Dr. Debbie Barker, Ph.D., CCC-SLP, University of
Central Oklahoma
Diane Bless, Ph.D., CCC-SLP, University of
Wisconsin-Madison
Gordon Blood, Ph.D., CCC-SLP, Pennsylvania State
University
Nancy Flores Castilleja, MA, CCC-SLP
Karen Chenausky, Speech Technology & Applied
Research
Ellen R. Cohn, Ph.D., CCC-SLP, University of
Pittsburg
Stephanie Davidson, Ph.D., CCC-A, Ohio State
University
Karen Beverly Ducker, ASHA Office of
Multicultural Affairs
Richard C. Folsom, Ph.D., CCC-A, University of
Washington-Seattle
Sybil Forsythe, MA, CCC-SLP
Vic S. Gladstone, Ph.D., CCC-A; Chief Staff Officer
for Audiology; Liaison to Academic Affairs,
Accreditation, Certification, & Ethics
Brian Goldstein, Ph.D., CCC-SLP, Temple University
Mary Jo Cooley Hidecker, MA, CCC-A/SLP,
Michigan State University
Erik Hein, former ASHA Director of Membership
Ceilia Hooper, MA, CCC-SLP, University of North
Carolina-Greensboro
Jeanne M. Johnson, Ph.D., CCC-SLP, Washington
State University
Ray Kent, Ph.D., CCC-SLP, University of Wisconsin-
Madison
Patricia B. Kricos, Ph.D., CCC-A, University of
Florida
Li-Rong Lilly Cheng, Ph.D., CCC-SLP, San Diego
State University
Mike Lynch, CCC-A, California State University

June McCullough, Ph.D., CCC-A, San Jose State
University
Claudia A. Magers, MS, CCC-SLP
Georgia McMann, ASHA Director of Certification
Administration
Malcolm R. McNeil, Ph.D., CCC-SLP, University of
Pittsburgh
Lemmietta G. McNeilly, Ph.D., CCC-SLP, Florida
International University
Arlene A. Pietranton, Ph.D., ASHA Executive
Director
Sandra Savinelli, SLPD, CCC-SLP, Nova
Southeastern University
Carol Scheffner Hammer, Ph.D., CCC-SLP,
Pennsylvania State University
Geralyn M. Schulz, Ph.D., CCC-SLP, George
Washington University
Neil T. Shepherd, Ph.D., CCC-A, University of
Pennsylvania
Staff of American Academy of Audiology (Ph.D.
in Hearing Sciences, Sc.D., and Au.D.
chapters)
Lillian N. Stiegler, Ph.D., CCC-SLP, Southeastern
Louisiana University
Nancy Swigert, MA, CCC-SLP
Candace Vickers, MS, CCC-SLP
Colleen F. Visconti, Ph.D., CCC-SLP, Baldwin-
Wallace College
Paige Wesley, ASHA Asset & Corporate Partner
Director
Laura Ann Wilber, Ph.D., CCC-SLP/A,
Northwestern University
Carol L. Williams, ASHA Certification Maintenance
Program Manager
Kenneth E. Wolf, Ph.D., CCC-A, Charles R. Drew
University of Medicine and Sciences
Heather Harris Wright, Ph.D., CCC-SLP, University
of Kentucky
Lisa Young, MS, CCC-A, University of Kentucky

## DELMAR LEARNING STAFF

Last, but certainly not least, NSSLHA expresses a big thank you to the Delmar Learning staff who spent many long hours assisting NSSLHA in getting this guide published.

Juliet Byington, Developmental Editor
Kalen Conerly, Acquisitions Editor
Jim Zayicek, Senior Production Editor

# CHAPTER 1

# Introduction to the Professions

## INTRODUCTION

A career in audiology and speech-language pathology is incredibly rewarding and exciting. These professionals positively impact the lives of individuals with communication challenges and their families by assessing, treating, and researching speech, language, and hearing disorders. Audiologists and speech-language pathologists can be certified as clinicians by the American Speech-Language-Hearing Association (ASHA) after completing academic course work, completing supervised clinical practicum hours, and passing the Praxis series examination in audiology or speech-language pathology that is administered by the Educational Testing Service (ETS). Additionally, individuals desiring ASHA certification in speech-language pathology must complete a mentored, 36-week Speech-Language Pathology Clinical Fellowship after graduation. Because speech and hearing work hand-in-hand, some professionals even choose to get degrees in both audiology and speech-language pathology.

When investigating degrees in communication sciences and disorders, it is important to understand how much education is needed to work professionally. Starting in 2012, entry-level audiologists must have a doctoral degree to be ASHA certified and to work in some states (currently, a minimum of a master's degree is required). In total, audiologists and speech-language pathologists who want to earn a master's degree go through six to eight years of higher education, including four to five years of undergraduate courses and two to three years of a graduate program. Audiologists and speech-language pathologists who obtain a doctorate will be in higher education for about eight to ten years (this includes four to five years of undergraduate courses and four to five years of a doctoral program). This chapter briefly examines the fields of audiology and speech-language pathology and is an excellent starting point for anyone interested in learning more about a degree in communication sciences and disorders.

# WHAT IS AUDIOLOGY?

• • • • • • • • • • • • • • • • • • • • • • • • • • •

Jeanette Glenn, master's student, audiology,
University of Wisconsin–Madison

*Audiology* is the study, diagnosis, treatment, and prevention of hearing and balance impairments. Audiologists are professionals trained to treat infants, children, and adults of all ages living with hearing loss. Audiology is an ideal career field for those who want to improve another person's quality of life by providing that person with greater access to hearing.

Audiology is an attractive career because it is so diverse. In addition to treating hearing loss, audiologists are responsible for dispensing hearing aids and developing treatments to prevent hearing loss. They work in the rehabilitation of persons with hearing and balance loss. Audiologists can also teach at a university, where they help students gain knowledge and obtain their degrees and certifications. Audiologists can be hearing scientists who engage in hearing research and design hearing equipment. There are many audiologists who are involved in a combination of these pursuits and may engage in research, clinical work, and instruction all at once. Within the field, there are many areas in which an audiologist can specialize, such as:

- **Auditory processing.** Auditory processing focuses on the peripheral and central auditory system manipulation of acoustic signals.

- **Auditory-verbal therapy.** This area focuses on identification, discrimination, recognition, and comprehension. An auditory-verbal therapist is an audiologist or speech-language pathologist who has been specially trained to provide caregivers (usually family members) of a person with a hearing impairment with the skills to use this therapy at home.

- **Cochlear implants.** Cochlear implants are hearing devices that are surgically implanted into the ear to improve hearing. The audiologist, in conjunction with a team of other medical professionals, is responsible for diagnosing the degree and type of hearing loss, assessing speech perception skills and tonal thresholds, and being actively involved in the rehabilitation of the patient's hearing throughout the process.

- **Educational audiology.** Specialists in this area conduct research and provide instruction.

- **Geriatric audiology.** This area involves diagnosing and providing appropriate rehabilitation for hearing loss among the elderly.

- **Intra-operative monitoring.** This involves monitoring a patient's hearing using electrophysiological testing during an operation.

- **Occupational audiology.** Occupational audiology involves preserving hearing in settings where there is possible harmful noise exposure, and studying the treatment and prevention of hearing loss and hearing conservation in industrial settings.

- **Pediatric audiology.** This area involves screening, diagnosing, and treating hearing loss in children. A pediatric audiologist also provides information on educational placements for children focusing on sign language and Deaf culture.

- **Vestibular disorders.** This area treats auditory nerve disorders affecting balance.

In addition to the many areas of specialization, audiologists work in a variety of different settings. Figure 1-1 provides a breakdown of the primary employment settings for ASHA-certified audiologists. These settings include:

- Corporations and non-profit organizations
- Colleges and universities
- Hospitals
- Private practice
- Rehabilitation clinics
- Schools

At the heart of the profession is each audiologist's desire to help the wide range of individuals with hearing and balance disorders and their families. Due to the great flexibility within the field, professionals can choose an area they truly enjoy. Regardless of which specialty, setting, or population an audiologist chooses to work with, every professional will be positively influencing another's life, making audiology an extremely rewarding career.

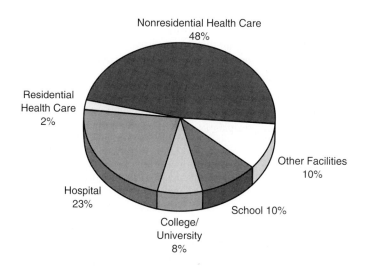

**Figure 1-1** ASHA-certified audiologists by primary employment facility
*(Source: ASHA Summary Membership and Affiliation Counts, 2003 year-end)*

# WHAT IS SPEECH-LANGUAGE PATHOLOGY?

Kelly Farquharson, master's student, SLP, Pennsylvania State University and NSSLHA Regional Councilor, Region 1, 2003–2005

Speech-Language Pathologists (SLPs), often called speech therapists or speech teachers, are the only professionals educated to assess, diagnose, and treat speech, language, and swallowing disorders. Because these activities are vital to the lives of every individual, imagine the impact on a life when at least one of these abilities is impaired. In a highly rewarding way, SLPs assist individuals with disorders of speech, language, and swallowing every day.

The field of speech-language pathology is suitable for individuals who wish to work with any age range, any special population, in any setting. The field is a wonderfully diverse and appealing career path to choose. Some of the most common areas of interest are:

- **Augmentative and alternative communication (AAC).** AAC provides a means of communication to individuals who are unable to independently and efficiently communicate verbally due to a limitation. Some examples of AAC include sign language and a portable computerized device with speech output.

- **Child language.** This area involves the examination of children's ability to properly formulate and express their thoughts into sentences. SLPs work to improve children's word choice, vocabulary, sentence structure, and social communication skills. They work with children who may say only a few or no words.

- **Cleft lip or palate.** This is a congenital condition involving a hole in the lip or in the hard or soft palate (the roof of a mouth). Cleft lip or palate causes a distortion of speech because it causes extra air flow from the mouth or nose. Because of this extra flow of air, individuals with cleft palate often sound "breathy" in that they are unable to control the outward flow of their air while talking.

- **Dysphagia.** This is a swallowing disorder caused by weakness in the muscles that are used to swallow, paralysis of the vocal folds, stroke (which can cause a paralysis of one part of the body), or other neurogenic disorder.

- **Fluency,** also known as **stuttering.** Fluency refers to the flow of speech and disfluency refers to the inability of speech to flow (as is seen in stuttering). This is an interesting field with ongoing research to determine the cause.

- **Neurogenic speech and language disorders.** These occur because of injury to the brain (before, during, or after birth). One common example of this often seen by SLPs is called aphasia, which is the inability to understand and/or express language.

- **Voice.** This involves working with impairments at the level of the larynx (e.g., the voice box or vocal chords) caused by misuse, neurogenic conditions, or external trauma.

These areas of interest are a mere overview and are by no means an exhaustive list of the areas of speech-language pathology. The possibilities are endless. This is similar for the settings in which an SLP can work. Figure 1-2 provides an overview of ASHA-Certified Speech-Language Pathologists by primary employment facility. Some of the settings where SLPs most commonly work in include:

- Acute care hospitals

- Charter schools

- Colleges and universities

- Corporations and non-profit organizations

- Nursing homes

- Private practices

- Rehabilitation hospitals

- Research labs

- Skilled nursing facilities

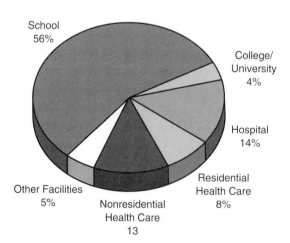

**Figure 1-2** ASHA-certified speech-language pathologists by primary employment facility *(Source: ASHA Summary Membership and Affiliation Counts, 2003 year-end)*

## CONCLUSION

As can be seen from the abundance of options for an audiologist or SLP, this career path can lead to a diverse professional life. The field is constantly changing and new research is always being conducted. This is very important to the practicing clinician, as the work being done by researchers today leads to new assessment and treatment options for individuals with communication disorders tomorrow. Within this field, anyone who wants to make a difference in the lives of others can find a niche in audiology or speech-language pathology.

# CHAPTER 2

# Job Outlook and Salary Expectations

Sherry L. Tracy, master's student, SLP, University of Wisconsin-Madison

## INTRODUCTION

One of the pressing concerns students have when choosing a major is whether it will lead to a job after graduation. For many students, it is important not only to do something enjoyable, but also to find a job that pays well. Certainly with the expense that goes into obtaining an undergraduate or graduate degree, it is important to know that, in the end, you will be able to achieve your personal goals and financially support yourself. This chapter discusses the job outlook for audiologists and speech-language pathologists (SLPs) and presents mean salaries for each profession. The good news is that for audiologists and SLPs, the job market looks very promising! As with most professions, an individual's earning potential depends on many factors, including personal motivation; area of specialization; where in the country you work; whether you work for a private practice, a not-for-profit clinic, or a research university; and how much you work (full-time, part-time, in an educational setting with summers off). While there are many variables, the mean salaries discussed in this chapter provide a good idea of the salary ranges to be expected.

## EMPLOYMENT OUTLOOK FOR AUDIOLOGY AND SPEECH-LANGUAGE PATHOLOGY

According to the *U.S. Department of Labor Bureau of Labor Statistics Occupational Outlook Handbook*, the future job outlook for audiology and speech-language pathology is promising. First of all, the elderly population is rapidly escalating. This is, in part, due to the baby boom generation reaching middle age and medical advances that have increased the survival rate of trauma and stroke victims. With the increasing elderly population and medical advances, employment opportunities in health and rehabilitation services are on the rise. For example, hearing loss is strongly associated with aging, so an aging population will create more jobs for audiologists. Likewise, as the older population grows, the incidence of cerebrovascular accidents (strokes) will likely rise, and the need for SLPs in rehabilitation clinics and hospitals will increase.

The growing need for the CSD professional is not limited to those working with aging populations. Employment of CSD professionals will increase as the public and health care professionals become more aware of the importance of identifying and diagnosing hearing, speech, and language problems early. Anticipated growth in elementary, secondary, and special education enrollments will create more employment of audiologists and SLPs in the schools. Special education and related services are guaranteed by federal law to all children who qualify (*Occupational Outlook Handbook*). This means there will be an increase in job opportunities for individuals interested in working with children who may have speech, language, and/or hearing challenges.

In addition, there is a rising use of contract services by schools, hospitals, and nursing facilities, as well as an increased demand for direct services to individuals. This will cause an increase in the number of audiologists and speech-language pathologists choosing to work in, or run, private practices. There is also a shortage of qualified personnel in inner cities, rural, and less populated areas of the country (*Fact Sheet: Speech-Language Pathology*). All this means more opportunities for individuals with CSD degrees.

In fact, over the next few years, it is expected that both professions of audiology and speech-language pathology will increase at a faster rate than average in comparison with all other occupations. An occupation report published by the U.S. Department of Labor Bureau of Labor Statistics shows that the occupation of audiology is expected to increase 29.0% and speech-language pathology is expected to increase 27.2% between 2002 and 2012. Other occupations will increase on an average of 14.8%. This report also shows a very low percentage of unemployed audiologists and SLPs.

A CSD professional's salary depends on his or her educational background, experience, area of specialty, type of worksetting, and geographical location (*Fact Sheet: Audiology*). In 2003, the median salary for audiologists was $55,000 for a calendar year. The median salary for SLPs was $52,600. See Figure 2-1 for the median annual salaries of audiologists from 1995 through

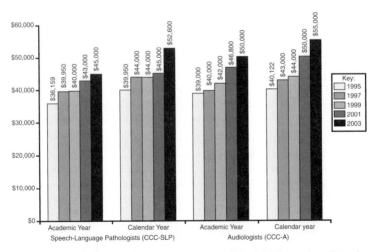

**Figure 2-1** Median annual salaries for ASHA-certified SLPs and audiologists, 1995-2003 (Calendar-year basis only) *(Adapted from ASHA 2003 Omnibus Survey)*

2003. The median starting salary for a calendar year basis was $43,000 for audiologists and $37,000 for SLPs. Figure 2-2 shows the median salaries based on academic and calendar years for audiologists and SLPs with a master's or doctorate degree. Figure 2-3 gives median salaries based on years of experience. Figure 2-4 shows median salaries based on geographic regions.

# Ph.D. SHORTAGE

Hearing, speech, and language scientists are research scientists who form the foundations of the fields of audiology and speech-language pathology by increasing or improving the knowledge base of these fields. These research scientists generally hold a Ph.D. in addition to the master's degree required to practice clinically. The job outlook is promising for these scientists. The field needs these researchers to:

- further investigate the neurophysiological, neurobiological, and physical processes that underlie normal communication.
- find new tools and techniques to prevent, identify, assess, and rehabilitate hearing, speech, and language impairments.
- examine the role of cultural diversity in human communication.
- explore causality and progression issues related to genetics and heredity.
- work with clinicians to design and implement both medical and behavioral treatment protocols for hearing, balance, speech, language, and swallowing disorders (*Fact Sheet: Speech, Language, & Hearing Science*).

There is a severe shortage of research scientists in CSD across the United States. In 1998, less than one percent of the 96,000 ASHA members and affiliates listed research as their primary function of employment (*Fact Sheet:*

| Salary Basis and Highest Degree | Certificate of Clinical Competence | | | | | | | |
|---|---|---|---|---|---|---|---|---|
| | (CCC-SLP) | | CCC-A | | CCC-SLP/A | | No CCC | |
| | Valid *n* | Median | Valid *n* | Median | Valid *n* | Median | Valid *n* | Median |
| **Academic year** | | | | | | | | |
| Master's | 692 | $45,000 | 101 | $47,000 | 93 | $48,400 | 120 | $37,313 |
| Doctorate | 13 | | 28 | $56,500 | 32 | $64,500 | 5 | |
| **Calendar year** | | | | | | | | |
| Master's | 327 | $52,000 | 550 | $52,000 | 86 | $63,500 | 70 | $40,000 |
| Doctorate | 12 | | $133 | $70,000 | 65 | $77,800 | 3 | |

**Figure 2-2** 2003 basic median annual salaries by salary basis, CCC status, and highest degree in profession(s) *(Adapted from ASHA 2003 Omnibus Survey)*

| Salary Basis, Number of Years Experience | Certificate of Clinical Competence | | | | | | | |
|---|---|---|---|---|---|---|---|---|
| | (CCC-SLP) | | CCC-A | | CCC-SLP/A | | No CCC | |
| | Valid *n* | Median | Valid *n* | Median | Valid *n* | Median | Valid *n* | Median |
| **Academic year** | | | | | | | | |
| 1–3 years | 89 | $37,000 | 7 | | 1 | | 98 | $36,715 |
| 4–6 years | 132 | $39,000 | 13 | | 4 | | 14 | |
| 7–9 years | 83 | $40,000 | | | 6 | | 4 | |
| 10–12 years | 68 | $45,000 | 34 | $45,000 | 5 | | 3 | |
| 13–15 years | 55 | $49,000 | | | 8 | | 1 | |
| 16–18 years | 43 | $49,000 | 29 | $50,000 | | | 2 | |
| 19–21 years | 66 | $53,000 | | | 28 | $49,808 | 0 | |
| 22–27 years | 116 | $52,000 | 50 | $57,000 | 29 | $53,000 | 3 | |
| 28 or more years | 62 | $60,000 | | | 49 | $62,000 | 5 | |
| **Calendar year** | | | | | | | | |
| 1–3 years | 59 | $42,000 | 120 | $43,000 | 2 | | 61 | $40,000 |
| 4–6 years | 62 | $47,250 | 100 | $50,000 | 5 | | 5 | |
| 7–9 years | 39 | $50,000 | 58 | $50,000 | 1 | | 0 | |
| 10–12 years | 33 | $55,000 | 60 | $53,900 | 1 | | 3 | |
| 13–15 years | 40 | $55,500 | 66 | $60,000 | 12 | | 0 | |
| 16–18 years | | | 52 | $63,500 | 6 | | 1 | |
| 19–21 years | 31 | $60,000 | 58 | $64,500 | 11 | | 0 | |
| 22–27 years | 40 | $64,800 | 96 | $70,500 | 34 | $67,000 | 0 | |
| 28 or more years | 43 | $68,500 | 84 | $77,000 | 72 | $80,000 | 5 | |

**Figure 2-3** 2003 basic median annual salaries by salary basis, CCC status, and number of years experience *(Adapted from ASHA Omnibus Survey, 2003)*

*Speech, Language, & Hearing Science*). In addition to research, individuals with doctorates in CSD can fill the important role of university faculty and professors who educate future students in the field. Currently, many faculty members are reaching retirement age, and there are not enough new Ph.D. candidates to fill their positions. In a survey of the Ph.D. programs, the mean age of Ph.D. faculty is 49 years. Across the U.S., there were 333 unfilled spots in Ph.D. programs (*Ph.D. Program Survey Results, 2002*). The employment prospects for individuals with doctoral degrees interested in performing research and teaching at a university are excellent.

For many, obtaining a doctoral degree can be a big financial commitment. However, based on a survey in 2002, 86% of CSD doctoral students received funding. There was a large range of funding granted to these students. The average levels were $14,730 for extramurally funded Ph.D. trainees or fellows; $13,550 for extramurally funded research assistants; $13,320 for university-funded research assistants; and $11,360 for university-funded teaching assistants.

| Salary Basis, Geographic Region, and Geographic Division | Certificate of Clinical Competence | | | | | | | |
|---|---|---|---|---|---|---|---|---|
| | (CCC-SLP) | | CCC-A | | CCC-SLP/A | | No CCC | |
| | Valid *n* | Median | Valid *n* | Median | Valid *n* | Median | Valid *n* | Median |
| Academic year | | | | | | | | |
| Northeast | 155 | $54,000 | 24 | | 36 | $60,750 | 31 | $43,000 |
| Middle Atlantic | 102 | $54,609 | 19 | | 30 | $61,250 | 23 | |
| New England | 53 | $50,199 | 5 | | 6 | | 8 | |
| Midwest | 200 | $44,000 | 43 | $50,000 | 30 | $53,000 | 26 | $34,391 |
| East North Central | 128 | $45,000 | 29 | $52,500 | 22 | | 19 | |
| West North Central | 72 | $40,000 | 14 | | 8 | | 7 | |
| South | 219 | $41,000 | 33 | $47,000 | 41 | $47,093 | 56 | $36,000 |
| East South Central | 35 | $36,000 | 3 | | 5 | | 5 | |
| South Atlantic | 117 | $42,000 | 25 | $47,000 | 20 | | 3 | $36,000 |
| West South Central | 67 | $40,000 | 5 | | 16 | | 18 | |
| West | 139 | $48,000 | 33 | $46,626 | 24 | | 17 | |
| Mountain | 57 | $43,150 | 16 | | 12 | | 8 | |
| Pacific | 82 | $52,550 | 17 | | 12 | | 9 | |

**U.S. Census Bureau geographic regions and divisions with corresponding states:**

| | | |
|---|---|---|
| **Northeast** | Middle Atlantic | New Jersey, New York, Pennsylvania |
| | New England | Connecticut, Maine, Massachusetts, New Hampshire, Rhode Island, Vermont |
| **Midwest** | East North Central | Illinois, Indiana, Michigan, Ohio, Wisconsin |
| | West North Central | Iowa, Kansas, Minnesota, Missouri, Nebraska, North Dakota, South Dakota |
| **South** | East South Central | Alabama, Kentucky, Mississippi, Tennessee |
| | South Atlantic | Delaware, District of Columbia, Florida, Georgia, Maryland, North Carolina, South Carolina, Virginia, West Virginia |
| | West South Central | Arkansas, Louisiana, Oklahoma, Texas |
| **West** | Mountain | Arizona, Colorado, Idaho, Montana, Nevada, New Mexico Utah, Wyoming |
| | Pacific | Alaska, California, Hawaii, Oregon, Washington |

**Figure 2-4** 2003 basic median annual salaries by salary basis, CCC status, and U. S. Census Bureau geographic regions and divisions *(Adapted from ASHA Omnibus Survey, 2003)*

Sixty-four percent of Ph.D. students received a full tuition waiver, while 19% received a partial waiver (*Ph.D. Program Survey Results, 2002*). The wide availability of funding, along with the excellent job market for individuals with a doctorate, are excellent news to individuals considering a doctorate in audiology or speech-language pathology.

You might wonder what the difference in earning potential is for individuals with a graduate degree and individuals with a doctorate. In 2003, the difference in median annual salary for individuals with a master's degree and those with a doctorate was $15,000 for audiologists and $10,114 for SLPs. The median salary for an audiologist with a Ph.D. was $70,000. For an SLP with a PhD, the median salary was $57,114 (*Occupational Outlook Handbook*). The median earning potential is higher for individuals with doctoral degrees, but it is important to remember that there are many other factors to be considered, including location, setting, and specialization.

## CONCLUSION

The data discussed in this chapter can be boiled down to a few important facts: people interested in helping individuals with communication and hearing challenges can look forward not only to making a positive impact on the lives of their clients, but they can expect to find rich opportunities in a healthy job market. In addition, according to reports on the median salary, they can expect to make a comfortable living.

## WORKS CITED

American Speech-Language-Hearing Association. *Fact Sheet: Audiology.* Rockville, MD, on the Internet at http://www.asha.org/students/professions/overview/audiology.htm (visited March 25, 2004).

American Speech-Language-Hearing Association. *Fact Sheet: Speech-Language Pathology.* Rockville, MD, on the Internet at http://www.asha.org/students/professions/overview/audiology.htm (visited March 25, 2004).

Bureau of Labor Statistics, U.S. Department of Labor. *Occupational Outlook Handbook, 2004–05 Edition, Audiologists,* on the Internet at http://www.bls.gov/oco/ocos085.htm (visited July 17, 2004).

Bureau of Labor Statistics, U.S. Department of Labor. *Occupational Outlook Handbook, 2004–05 Edition, Speech-Language Pathologists,* on the Internet at http://www.bls.gov/oco/ocos099.htm (visited July 17, 2004).

Janota, J. (2004, Feb. 3). Annual, hourly salary figures available: Salary results of the 2003 ASHA Omnibus Survey released. *The ASHA Leader,* pp. 1–10.

# CHAPTER 3

# The National Student Speech Language Hearing Association

Dawn D. Dickerson, MPA, NSSLHA Director of Operations

## INTRODUCTION

The National Student Speech Language and Hearing Association (NSSLHA) is a pre-professional membership association for students interested in the study of communication sciences and disorders (CSD). NSSLHA averages 12,000 members and has 300 local chapters at colleges and universities throughout the United States, Canada, and Greece. Students can separately apply for membership to NSSLHA at the local and national levels. To clearly distinguish references to local versus national, NSSLHA always refers to the national association or national level membership.

## THE PURPOSE OF NSSLHA

NSSLHA exists to provide students interested in the field of CSD with a closer affiliation to professionals in the discipline. A student that chooses membership in NSSLHA is making an investment in becoming a better CSD professional. NSSLHA members learn, early in their careers, the value of advocacy, certification, continuing education, ethics, and research in contributing to their long-term success. NSSLHA is a student-run association, independent of the professional association, the American Speech-Language-Hearing Association (ASHA). The national association is governed by an Executive Council (EC) that consist of ten NSSLHA members (students), who serve as Regional Councilors (RCs), and five ASHA members (faculty), who serve as consultants to the Council. Issues that affect students or the operation of the association are brought before the EC. The council is responsible for discussing those issues and determining a solution or course of action in the best interest of the majority of the membership.

Any student, full- or part-time, undergraduate or graduate, national or international, may apply for membership in NSSLHA. You may join NSSLHA even if there is not a chapter at your college or university. NSSLHA membership is not available to a student who has applied for the Certificate of Clinical

Competence from the American Speech-Language-Hearing Association. Figure 3-1 lists the top ten benefits of membership in NSSLHA.

Joining the national association is easy:

- Complete the membership application provided on the last two pages of this guide.
- Visit http://www.nsslha.org/join and download a membership application.
- Call the ASHA Action Center at 800-498-2071 and enroll over the phone with a major credit card (Mastercard or Visa only).
- Ask the NSSLHA chapter at your university for an application and mail in your application with check, money order, or credit card information to NSSLHA, 10801 Rockville Pike, Rockville, MD 20852.

1. Eligibility for the NSSLHA-to-ASHA Conversion Program Discount. Students with two consecutive years of membership in NSSLHA immediately prior to graduation receive a significant discount on the initial dues and fees for ASHA membership and certification.

2. Two issues of *Contemporary Issues in Communication Science and Disorders (CICSD)*, a NSSLHA journal.

3. Three issues of NSSLHA's newsletter, *News & Notes*.

4. The *ASHA Leader*, an ASHA newspaper about issues related to the professions.

5. A print subscription to one of the following ASHA journals: *American Journal of Audiology; American Journal of Speech-Language Pathology; Journal of Speech, Language, and Hearing Research;* or *Language, Speech, and Hearing Services in Schools*.

6. Access to the "members only" areas of the NSSLHA and ASHA Web sites, which include all ASHA journals (full-text), ASHA's Literature Review Service, advocacy, and convenient membership dues renewal.

7. Technical assistance and resources from ASHA professional staff.

8. Preference for special offers, scholarships, grants, and programs for CSD students through NSSLHA and ASHA.

9. Professional liability, medical, and dental insurance through plans available exclusively to NSSLHA members.

10. A reduced registration fee for the ASHA convention.

**Figure 3-1** The top ten NSSLHA membership benefits

You can also join your local NSSLHA chapter, which is different from being a member of the national association (and dues are separately paid). Local chapters organize fun activities that allow you to meet other students who share your interest in CSD. Most chapters provide community service projects and have speakers at some of their meetings. Attending meetings and events provides an opportunity to speak with classmates to discuss courses and provide encouragement. Being an active NSSLHA chapter member looks good on graduate school applications and resumés (e.g., where you can list community service activities and leadership positions).

To join your chapter, contact the local NSSLHA chapter president or chapter advisor in your department for information about dues and meetings. A list of NSSLHA chapters with links to chapter presidents and Web sites is available on the NSSLHA Web site at http://www.nsslha.org.

## CONCLUSION

To get up-to-date information on leadership opportunities, scholarships, and conventions and conferences, go to the NSSLHA Web site at http://www.nsslha.org. Contact your NSSLHA Regional Councilor when you have questions related to the field. If he or she does not know the answers, you will be directed to someone who does.

# CHAPTER 4

# Financing Your CSD Education

Kristi L. Pennypacker, master's student, SLP at Bloomsburg University of Pennsylvania and Marie Patton, master's student, SLP, University of Wisconsin-Madison and NSSLHA President, 2002–2003*

## INTRODUCTION

If you are like most students, you probably cannot afford to pay for college and graduate school by yourself. Fortunately, the government, independent agencies, and educational institutions offer a wide range of financial aid and scholarship opportunities. This chapter explains how to apply for federal student loans, what is usually required for scholarships, useful Web sites, and scholarships available through the American Speech-Language-Hearing Foundation (ASHF). While it does take some initiative on your part to seek out and apply for scholarships and financial aid, the return on this investment of time and energy can be significant.

## HOW TO SEEK FINANCIAL AID THROUGH THE GOVERNMENT

The federal government is an excellent place to begin looking for financial aid. As with most financial aid opportunities, it is your responsibility to seek out what is available and to follow through to maximize your chance for success. Figure 4-1 provides a checklist of steps to begin this process and the following section goes into detail about each of these steps.

☐ Complete the Free Application for Federal Student Aid (FAFSA).

☐ Consider a Stafford Loan.

☐ Visit the financial aid office at your college.

☐ Keep copies of the financial aid forms.

**Figure 4-1**  Obtaining government-sponsored financial aid

*Kristi worked in a financial aid office for over three years, and Marie has obtained various forms of financial support.*

# Complete the Free Application for Federal Student Aid

The Free Application for Federal Student Aid (FAFSA) is a report used by the university financial aid office to determine a student's eligibility for federal aid regardless of his or her financial status. The FAFSA must be filled out each year that a student is applying for financial aid. The form can be completed online at http://www.fafsa.ed.gov or a paper version is available through the university financial aid office. The FAFSA must be completed for consideration for a Pell Grant and the Stafford Loan. Only undergraduate students are eligible for the federally funded Pell Grants. These grants do not need to be repaid and are awarded based on income (contact your financial aid office for more information). Stafford Loans are discussed in greater detail in the next section. Deadlines for the FAFSA vary for different states, so refer to the schedule of deadlines listed on the FAFSA Web site or check with your financial aid office.

When completing the FAFSA, it is helpful to have your current tax documents available. If you are a dependent on your parents' tax return, you will also need your parents' tax documents. Keep in mind that most financial aid is distributed on a first-come, first-served basis. It is important to apply early. Do not let the fact that you do not have tax information readily available keep you from submitting an application. You can always answer the financial questions based on estimates and update the information later.

It takes two to three weeks for electronically submitted applications to be processed and four to six weeks for paper applications to be processed. For electronic applications, you will receive an email and a letter in the mail detailing your eligibility. If you mail in the form, a Student Aid Report (SAR) will be mailed back to you verifying the information from the FAFSA form. You must review this report and make any necessary corrections. Once you receive a letter detailing your eligibility, your university's financial aid office will send you information regarding the amount of money you are eligible to receive and a promissory note to complete.

It is important to note that the summer starts a new school year. Thus, the FAFSA form for 2006-2007 will cover the summer 2006, fall 2006, and spring 2007 semesters. However, you should check with the college that you are attending to make sure they define a school year the same as stated above.

## Consider a Stafford Loan

The FAFSA form asks if the student is interested in a student loan. If marked yes, the federal government will automatically send a Stafford Loan application. The Stafford Loan is available to all students, undergraduate and graduate, and payment does not begin on this loan until six months after the student graduates or withdraws from the university. The six-month grace period begins if a student's enrollment drops below the university's part-time credits per semester. If a student decides to return to school, his or her loans can be deferred again so that the payments are not required while he or she is at least half time in school. The loans can be repaid early without any penalties.

The two types of Stafford Loans are subsidized and unsubsidized. With subsidized Stafford Loans, the interest does not have to be paid by the student while he or she is in school. However, unsubsidized loans require that the interest be paid while the student is in school, or the student can contact his or her lender to see if the interest can be capitalized and added to the total after graduation. The subsidized Stafford Loan is need-based and the federal government sets the standards. The loan amounts are for the whole school year, and at the time of publication, undergraduate students can borrow up to $2,625 for year one; $3,500 for year two; $5,500 per year for years three and four; and graduate students can borrow $8,500 per year. The unsubsidized Stafford Loan is not need-based. The amounts that a student can borrow in unsubsidized Stafford Loans were taken from Sallie Mae at http://www. salliemae.com/apply/borrowing/stafford.html. Year one: $2,625 (dependent student) and $6,625 (independent student); year two: $3,500 (dependent) and $7,500 (independent); years three and four: $5,500 per year (dependent) and $10,500 per year (independent). Graduate students can borrow up to $18,500 per year minus the amount of any subsidized Stafford Loan processed for them.

There are limits on the amount of cumulative Stafford Loans that students can borrow as well. At the time of publication, according to Sallie Mae, if the student is considered a dependent student and is an undergraduate, then he or she can borrow up to $23,000 (combined subsidized and unsubsidized) and up to $46,000 if the student is an independent undergraduate student ($23,000 of this total can be subsidized). Graduate students can borrow a total of $138,500 and $65,500 can be a subsidized Stafford Loan (http://www.salliemae.com/apply/borrowing/stafford.html).

If there is a reduction in a family's income due to a loss of a job, medical illness, or parental separation or divorce, etc., a student can call the university's financial aid office and ask for a Special Conditions form, which will take these income differences into account when determining aid eligibility. Any questions regarding the Stafford Loan can be directed to the college's financial aid office or to the higher education assistance agency in your state (http://www.aessuccess.org).

## Visit the Financial Aid Office at Your College

Avoid confusion and frustration when completing financial aid applications by going to the university's financial aid office and making an appointment with a financial aid advisor or supervisor. Take the FAFSA form and your 1040 and W2 forms (including your parents' if you are still a dependent) to your appointment, along with a list of any questions you may have. Other tax forms may be required if your family owns their own business or receives social security benefits. If you are unsure of what is needed, call ahead to get a list of the necessary forms and documents. Do not let your frustration at this process discourage you. The financial aid office is there to help you through this often confusing paperwork.

## Keep Copies of the Financial Aid Forms

Keep copies of everything! When filling out these same forms next year, you can go back and look at which lines on your tax forms correspond to questions on the FAFSA. By filling out the FAFSA accurately, some of the additional paperwork will be reduced, as no correction will be necessary. It is a good idea to keep copies of your financial aid forms for at least a year after you graduate. If you are paying back loans and have questions, you may need to refer to the original paperwork.

# HOW TO SEEK AND OBTAIN SCHOLARSHIPS AND GRANTS

Scholarships are a great way to help you afford school. The only catch is that you need to know what scholarships are available and then be an ideal applicant. Many scholarships require you to write one or more essays, list your GPA and activities, and have at least one letter of recommendation. Again, to benefit from these opportunities, it is up to you to be persistent and diligent. There are many different scholarships available based on a wide range of criteria, and with the considerable investment you are making in your education, it is in your best interest to investigate these options. The additional financial support of a scholarship can really help you focus on getting the most out of your education. Figure 4-2 is a checklist for seeking and obtaining scholarships and the following section goes into detail about each of the steps.

## Actively Hone Your Writing Skills

Many scholarships require essays and do not have interviews. Thus, the main way for scholarship reviewers to get to know you is to read a sample of your writing. Scholarship reviewers usually like applicants who exhibit strong writing skills. However, your content is just as important as the structure and clarity of your writing.

Many scholarships have topics such as, "Why do you feel that you deserve this scholarship?", "What school/community activities you have been involved with?", "What are your goals for the future?" It is important that you are careful to always answer the questions asked. It can be very easy to go off on a tangent. If you do not provide the decision-makers with the information they need to make a good decision, you can hurt your chances. Also, pay close attention to any formatting or style requirements. If the scholarship application requires you to provide a double-spaced, typed essay, do not hurt your chances by giving them a single-spaced, handwritten essay. When you write

- [ ] Actively hone your writing skills.
- [ ] Maintain a high grade point average (GPA) to be competitive.
- [ ] Be involved in organizations and keep track of your achievements.
- [ ] Build a good rapport with your professors.
- [ ] Avoid scholarships from companies that charge application fees.
- [ ] Ask for a list of scholarships at your financial aid office.
- [ ] Ask your academic advisor about department scholarships.
- [ ] Build relationships with administrative people in the CSD department and financial aid office.
- [ ] Visit the Web site of your state speech-language-hearing association.
- [ ] Find out about available graduate assistantships.
- [ ] Contact the financial aid office for information on work-study positions.
- [ ] Visit the American Speech-Language-Hearing Foundation (ASHF) Web site.
- [ ] Visit other Web sites for financial aid resources.
- [ ] Purchase *Funding Sources* from ASHA.
- [ ] Keep searching and applying for scholarships.

**Figure 4-2** Checklist for obtaining scholarships and grants

scholarship essays, always have a peer review your essay before submission to check for grammatical errors and clarity. If your campus has a writing center, it is an excellent idea to make an appointment to have someone skilled in editing review your work. You can also ask a trusted teacher, professor, or advisor to read over your work. To scholarship reviewers, the essay is a reflection of who you are. Put forth your best effort and really shine!

## Maintain a High Grade Point Average (GPA) to Be Competitive

Most scholarships want to know your GPA to ensure that you are in good academic standing. Keep your GPA up by seeking help from your professors and peers when you have questions, studying your notes regularly, taking a study skills course, reading your textbooks and completing homework assignments, attending classes, and forming study groups. GPAs of 3.0 or higher are usually needed for consideration of smaller scholarships, and 3.5 or higher is needed for larger scholarships. However, do not be afraid to apply for a scholarship just because you think everyone else will have a 4.0 GPA (and especially do not be afraid to apply if you have a 4.0). Since applications for some scholarships can take some time, not everyone who is eligible applies.

Read through scholarship applications carefully and identify what materials are needed to verify you are a student. You will probably have to order an official transcript from your university registrar's office. Depending on your school, there may be a fee for this. Contact your registrar's office if you have questions.

## Be Involved in Organizations and Keep Track of Your Achievements

Gain experience and knowledge in the field by joining academic, service, or community organizations, such as NSSLHA. In addition to rewarding academic and social experiences, being a member of an organization provides participation, involvement, and/or educational resources (e.g., journals) that many scholarship committees consider. Scholarship committees typically want to know if you have been awarded any special honors, such as the Dean's List, or awards through your department.

## Build a Good Rapport with Your Professors

Get to know your professors by asking them questions during lectures or make appointments to meet with them individually. Professors usually like students who are inquisitive and active participants in their education. Getting to know your professors not only helps you learn more from your courses, but it gives you the opportunity to find mentors who may help you grow into a better student, clinician, teacher, and/or researcher.

Most scholarships require letters of recommendation from at least one professor in your field who can describe your work ethic and academic achievements. Always ask a professor if he or she is willing to write you a *positive* letter of recommendation. You definitely do not want a professor to write you a negative one! Sometimes it is easiest to ask the professor in a letter or an email if he or she has time to write you a positive letter. Asking a professor in person, especially one you do not have a close relationship with, may be uncomfortable. Give anyone writing a recommendation for you plenty of time to complete the letter. Do not wait until the last minute! If someone has agreed to put the time and thought into writing a recommendation for you, it is common courtesy for you to give them ample time to complete the letter.

Once a professor agrees, provide the following in a neat packet (e.g., large envelope):

- a copy of the recommendation form or the writing prompt(s)
- an up-to-date resumé or list of activities

- a stamped and preaddressed envelope (if the letter needs to be mailed)
- a note (e.g., sticky note) to remind the professor of the due date and full name of the scholarship (which the professor will probably want to mention when writing the letter), and a thank you for taking the time to write the letter of recommendation

After the professor writes you the letter, send a thank-you card. After you hear about the scholarship (especially if you get it), make sure you share the hopefully good news.

## Avoid Scholarships from Companies That Charge Application Fees

Many students have reported getting letters in the mail or via email from organizations that claim to help find scholarships for a fee. It is difficult to know if the organization is credible. Before sending anyone money, check out their organization thoroughly. If you cannot track them down to ask questions, or if things seem a little too good to be true, walk away. As with any solicitation received via email or online, do not give out your credit card number without verifying that the company is legitimate.

## Ask for a List of Scholarships at Your Financial Aid Office

Contact your financial aid office for scholarship information pertinent to your school and your major. Lists are often available according to majors or colleges.

## Ask Your Academic Advisor About Department Scholarships

Your academic advisor is an excellent resource. In addition to being a potential mentor or someone to write a recommendation, advisors tend to have updated information about scholarships and awards offered through the department. Often scholarships are set up by alumni or former professors just for individuals in a particular major. Also check your department's Web site or check with the department chairperson for scholarship information.

## Build Relationships with Administrative People in the CSD Department and Financial Aid Office

Get to know the support staff in your department, as well as in the financial aid office. Often secretaries, administrative assistants, and other individuals who work in your department may have up-to-date information about scholarships, assistantships, and other opportunities. They are an invaluable resource.

# Visit the Web Site of Your State Speech-Language-Hearing Association

Some state associations offer student scholarships. To take advantage of these opportunities, you must be a member of your state association. Learn more about these opportunities by linking to state association Web sites available on the student resources page of http://www.nsslha.org.

## Find Out About Available Graduate Assistantships

Many universities rely on graduate students to help professors with research projects or their undergraduate teaching responsibilities. Depending on the university and the program, there may be a variety of graduate assistantships available (e.g., research, teaching, clinical, and project). In exchange for the graduate student's work, some assistantships offer a tuition waiver and/or a monetary stipend. For example, for a particular program, a graduate student may commit to assisting a professor with a research project for 15 to 20 hours a week for an academic year. In exchange, that student might receive a waiver of all costs of tuition. In another program, a graduate student may assist a professor with one undergraduate class per semester and receive a monetary stipend of $500 per semester. Check with your program to see what is available and what kind of time commitment may be required. This can be an excellent way to offset the cost of your graduate education, while gaining unique experiences from a professor.

## Contact the Financial Aid Office for Information on Work-Study Positions

Often a university offers a work-study program for both undergraduate and graduate students. Work-study positions involve working in an office or facility on campus. Try to locate a work-study position close to your area of professional interest. This will allow you earn money and gain valuable work experience that will increase your knowledge and give you an experience to list on your resumé.

## Visit the American Speech-Language-Hearing Foundation (ASHF) Web Site

Go to http://www.ashfoundation.org to download scholarship applications for students in CSD. The Foundation currently offers the following student scholarships:

- **Graduate Student Scholarship**

  You can apply for a Graduate Student Scholarship if you are a full-time graduate student in CSD or if you are a senior-level college student who has been accepted into a graduate program.

  Award: $4,000

- **Minority Student Scholarship**

  You can apply for a Minority Student Scholarship if you are an ethnic student who is a citizen of the United States and has been accepted into a graduate program.

  Award: $4,000

- **Student with a Disability Scholarship**

  You can apply for a Student with a Disability Scholarship if you are a graduate student with a disability who is enrolled or accepted in CSD graduate program.

  Award: $2,000

- **International/Minority Student Scholarship**

  You can apply for an International/Minority Student Scholarship if you are a full-time international/minority graduate student studying CSD in the United States.

  Award: $4,000

## Visit Other Web Sites for Financial Aid Resources

Following is a list of additional Web sites containing information about financial aid resources (retrieved March 8, 2004, from http://www.bloomu.edu/aid/index.php):

- U.S. Department of Education at http://www.ed.gov
- FSA Ombudsman at http://ombudsman.ed.gov/ombudsman/index.html
- Upromise-The Way to Save for College at http://www.upromise.com
- Tuition Pay at https://secure.tuitionpay.com

## Purchase *Funding Sources* from ASHA

AHSA's *Funding Sources: A Guide for Future Audiologists, Speech-Language Pathologists and Speech, Language and Hearing Scientists* gives detailed information about local, state, and national funding opportunities for all CSD students. You can obtain information about ordering this publication from the ASHA Products Catalog at http://www.asha.org.

# Keep Searching and Applying for Scholarships

Some students put a lot of effort into applying for scholarships in their first year or two, but do not continue to pursue these opportunities later in their college career. Do not be discouraged if you have not received a scholarship. Try again next year. Some scholarships prefer to give scholarships to those who have applied in previous years, and did not receive it. Other scholarships have preferences for older students (e.g., second year master's students over first years), but do not advertise the preference. If you do not apply for a scholarship, you definitely will not get it; so, take a chance and apply if the scholarship seems credible.

## CONCLUSION

Learning about the types of loans and grants from the government and researching scholarships is your first step toward paying for your education. You must be certain to follow the directions explicitly on applications for loans, grants, and scholarships. Also, essays for scholarships need to be well written, since many scholarship committees do not have an interview process, and your writing sample is one way that they get to know an applicant. Many options are available for financial aid, you just need to take advantage of the opportunities.

# CHAPTER 5

# The Importance of Shared Audiology and Speech-Language Pathology Courses

## INTRODUCTION

When undergraduates begin their required coursework in CSD, they are likely to wonder why they share the same major with students who have different career goals. Usually during undergraduate coursework, audiology students take some SLP-oriented courses. Likewise, SLP students take some audiology-oriented courses. It is not until graduate school when students begin to specialize their studies. Although audiology and speech-language pathology are different fields, there is considerable overlap. Both audiologists and SLPs assess, diagnose, and treat individuals with communication disorders.

## WHY SHARE COURSEWORK?

Some of the reasons why future audiologists and speech-language pathologists share the same coursework include:

- **Hearing, speech, and language are intricately related.** Audiologists and SLPs need a comprehensive understanding of human development, anatomy, and the communication process.

- **Clients who have certain conditions that are treated by audiologists may have speech and/or language disorders.** An audiologist may work with children with receptive language disorders. An audiologist who has a background in speech and language will be able to understand a client's needs and adjust his or her language so that the child will understand the tasks. Speech-language pathologists may see clients who have a hearing loss and/or auditory processing disorders. SLPs who work with older adults with voice, swallowing, speech, and/or language disorders are likely to have clients with hearing loss due to normal aging. As a result, SLPs may refer their clients to audiologists to assess their hearing.

- **On multidisciplinary teams, audiologists and SLPs work together in evaluating clients.** It is helpful to know more about other professionals' scopes of practice when you interact with them.

- **CSD professionals work together with individuals who are candidates for cochlear implants.** Audiologists complete evaluations for the implant, and SLPs teach speech to clients after the implantation.
- **SLPs need to rule out hearing loss as a possible cause or factor to a client's speech or language disorder.** An SLP may have difficulty providing treatment to a child or adult with an untreated hearing loss. The client is likely to struggle in understanding the SLP without a hearing aid, sign language, or other adaptive strategies that may be recommended by an audiologist. An SLP should be competent in basic hearing screening.
- **SLPs should have a background in knowing how hearing aids work.** SLPs are likely to work with clients with a hearing aid and should know how to replace a battery and adjust the volume in some hearing aid models.

These are just a few reasons why the fields of audiology and speech-language pathology share coursework at the undergraduate level. As you continue your study in the profession, you will discover more ways the professions are interrelated.

## WORKING TOGETHER TO IMPROVE EFFECTIVENESS

The following list provides some suggestions on how future audiologists and SLPs can work together to improve the effectiveness of treatment given to clients.

- If you are an audiologist who has a child client with a hearing impairment, screen your client's speech and language and/or refer the child to an SLP. If you are an SLP, screen your client's hearing and/or refer your client to an audiologist.
- If you are an audiologist who is seeing an adult who had a stroke, suffered traumatic brain injury (TBI), or other neurological deficiencies, consider referring the adult to an SLP, based on what you know about characteristics of speech and language disorders. If you are an SLP who has an adult client with TBI, aphasia, or other neurological deficits, consider referring the client to an audiologist, based on what you know about characteristics of hearing loss.
- If you are an audiologist, know at least one SLP who works with children and adult clients. You can contact the SLP when you have pertinent questions about a client with a speech and/or language disorder. If you are an SLP, know at least one audiologist who works in diagnostics and aural rehabilitation. You can contact the audiologist when a client has a possible hearing loss or you are uncertain about a type of aural rehabilitation treatment.
- Lobby Congress about bills that will affect your professions and shared clients. ASHA members have access to the advocacy Web page that lists current legislative issues Congress is considering related to these professions.

Contact information for Congresspersons is also listed. Visit the Legislation and Advocacy page of the ASHA Web site regularly and stay informed about the issues impacting the professions. Advocacy is key to ensuring that our careers and clients are protected.

## CONCLUSION

Audiologists and SLPs share more than coursework and the common goal of helping individuals with communication disorders. The American Speech-Language-Hearing Association currently accredits colleges and universities through the Council of Academic Accreditation on Audiology and Speech-Language Pathology. To be an ASHA-certified audiologist, students must currently complete clinical clock hours in speech/language screening. To be an ASHA-certified SLP, students must currently complete clinical clock hours in aural rehabilitation and hearing screening. This large professional organization provides certification, continuing education, support, and services to individuals working in both fields, thus furthering the close association between audiologists and SLPs that begins with shared undergraduate coursework and continues through to professional practice.

# CHAPTER 6

# Advice for High School Students

## INTRODUCTION

If you are a high school student interested in a career in audiology or speech-language pathology, this chapter will guide you through what you can do before you start college. Read on for tips on how to really figure out if this is the career path for you, how to prepare for college, and how to find a college with a major for audiologists and SLPs. Figure 6-1 provides a handy checklist of things to do to help you prepare for this next step.

☐ Learn more about what audiologists and SLPs do.

☐ Job shadow a local audiologist, SLP, or speech-language-hearing scientist.

☐ Keep track of hours you spend observing an audiologist or SLP.

☐ Keep your science notes.

☐ Take courses in science that will prepare you for college.

☐ Take writing courses.

☐ Make sure the colleges/universities you apply to have a Communication Science and Disorders (CSD) program.

☐ Visit a National Student Speech Language Hearing Association (NSSLHA) chapter.

☐ Visit the CSD department where you are applying to college.

☐ Order a complimentary subscription to NSSLHA's newsletter.

☐ Get involved.

☐ Consider working part-time.

☐ Volunteer.

**Figure 6-1** Checklist for high school students interested in a Communication Sciences and Disorders undergraduate degree

# Learn More About What Audiologists and SLPs Do

To make informed decisions about where you want to go to school and what you want to spend your time studying, learn as much as you can about the profession. Most libraries have books about health care professions, such as Stanfield, P.P. and Hui, Y. H. *Introduction to the Healthcare Professions, 3rd ed.*, Jones & Bartlett Publishers, Inc. (1998). You may also find books about sign language, Deaf culture, disabilities, hearing loss, stuttering, autism, hearing aids, and other topics related to communication disorders. Spending some time at your local library can really help you understand what a career in communication sciences and disorders could mean for you. If you like to read, there are a number of excellent novels and guidebooks related to CSD available. See Appendix C for suggestions.

Another great place to learn more about the profession is online. Visit the Student section of the NSSLHA Web site at http://www.nsslha.org and the student section of the ASHA Web site at http://www.asha.org and search for current issues in the professions.

# Job Shadow a Local Audiologist, SLP, or Speech-Language-Hearing Scientist

Job shadowing provides an opportunity for a student to follow a professional during a typical day at work. By job shadowing, you get to see first hand what the typical day of a professional is like. This is a great way to help you decide if a career in audiology or speech-language pathology is really right for you.

Audiologists and SLPs work in various settings, including hospitals; speech and hearing clinics; and elementary, middle, and high schools. To locate an audiologist or SLP, look in the phone book for a clinical practice, call a local hospital and ask to speak with the audiologist or speech-language pathologist, or contact your guidance office and ask if your school district has an audiologist or SLP on staff or on call. You can also ask family members and friends if they know of anyone who works professionally as an audiologist or SLP. Sometimes a personal reference can help you get your foot in the door.

When you speak with the audiologist or SLP over the phone, you may want to say the following: "I am a student at _____ High School. I am interested in becoming an audiologist/speech-language pathologist. If you have time, I would like to come in to briefly talk with you about the profession and to possibly observe your day at work."

When you observe the audiologist or SLP, dress professionally. Wear a nice pair of pants and a dress shirt or sweater. Dressing in jeans and a T-shirt would be inappropriate for most settings. Ask the audiologist or SLP what you should wear. Depending on the setting, there may be a specific dress code that you will need to observe. It is important to be respectful of the individual you are meeting with and the patients or clients you may come in contact with. If someone has kindly agreed to take time out of their busy work day to meet with you, the impression you make can influence his or her decision to meet with other high school students interested in job shadowing.

To make the most of your time with the audiologist or SLP, you should prepare questions ahead of time and bring a pen and notebook to take notes. Some questions you may want to ask include:

- What do you do here? What's a typical day like?
- What do you like best about your job?
- What do you find to be the most challenging part of your job?
- Have you worked in a different setting? What do you like about the settings you have worked in? What have you not liked?
- What advice do you have for a student who is interested in this profession?

After you meet with or observe the audiologist or SLP, be sure to send a thank-you note. While a thank-you email is thoughtful, an actual thank-you note received via mail makes a much better impression. If you are interested in continuing your research into the field, mention that you would be interested in volunteering. Ask if the audiologist or SLP knows of any opportunities. You want to establish good relationships early. If you have the opportunity to work as a volunteer with a professional, you may want to call on him or her in the future for a reference or a letter of recommendation.

## Keep Track of Hours You Spend Observing an Audiologist or SLP

Some undergraduate programs may be interested in learning that you have logged some observation hours with an audiologist or SLP. Your time observing while in high school can give you a jump on your preparation for the professions. Keep in mind that the hours observed in high school are separate from the observation hours required for ASHA certification. The observation hours required by ASHA will probably be addressed in your undergraduate program during your junior and/or senior years. For your personal information, keep a folder, binder, or computer record of all the time you spend observing an audiologist or SLP. You should also keep contact information of all individuals you observed or volunteered with. Be sure to have their name, address, phone number, email address, and the name of their practice, company, hospital, or employer.

## Keep Your Science Notes

Many of the research practices that you learn in biology and anatomy classes are reintroduced in college-level communication science classes. Pay attention! You will need this information in the future.

# Take Courses in Science That Will Prepare You for College

If your school offers Advanced Placement courses, consider taking biology, chemistry, and/or physics. These courses are not a requirement, but you will be surprised to find that some of the concepts you learn in these courses are reintroduced in undergraduate and graduate courses. With all that you will be learning in your undergraduate coursework, it can help you feel more comfortable and successful if you have a good background in science.

## Take Writing Courses

Any courses that strengthen your writing skills will be extremely useful. Find out if your high school offers a rhetoric or an advanced grammar course and take it if possible. You will use your writing skills frequently during your undergraduate and graduate coursework, so focusing on developing them will pay off when you are writing term papers, observation reports, and possibly a thesis. Having excellent writing skills is also helpful when writing essays for scholarships and admittance into academic programs. Make it easier on yourself by becoming a good writer now. Try to think like an English teacher when you write. Make a list of feedback that your teacher makes on your English papers so that you learn from your mistakes, such as using active voice instead of passive voice. The more you write, the easier the process will become and the more proficient you will be. Take advantage of any opportunity you have to practice your writing skills and to get constructive feedback on your work.

## Make Sure the Colleges/Universities You Apply to Have a Communication Science and Disorders (CSD) Program

Not all universities and colleges have a CSD program. Look on the university or college Web sites and search under key words, such as audiology, speech-language pathology, and communication disorders. Depending on the program, the department is sometimes called Communication Disorders and Sciences, Communication Disorders, or Communicative Disorders. You can also go to the Council for Academic Programs in Communication Sciences and Disorders (CAPCSD) Web site at http://www.capcsd.org or the National Association of Pre-Professional Programs (NAPP) Web site at http://www. napp.org for colleges and universities that have CSD programs.

## Visit a National Student Speech Language Hearing Association (NSSLHA) Chapter

To learn more about undergraduate coursework in CSD and to talk with students about their experience, visit a local college or university chapter of the

National Student Speech Language Hearing Association. To find a chapter in your state, go to the chapter section of the NSSLHA Web site at http://www. nsslha.org. Call the university's communication sciences and disorders department (which may also be called communication disorders and sciences, or communicative disorders). Ask for the NSSLHA chapter advisor. Explain to the chapter advisor that you are a high school student and, with permission, would like to sit in on the next NSSLHA meeting. Ask for the date, time and location. Then ask for the chapter president's email address, let him or her know that you will come, and would like to talk with him or her after the meeting about the department. Have a list of prepared questions, as well as a pen and notebook to take notes. Be sure to thank the chapter president or any other students for taking the time to meet with you. It would be a good idea to also send a thank you email to let them know you appreciate their help.

## Visit the CSD Department Where You Are Applying to College

Visiting the schools you are applying to is an excellent way to determine if the campus is the right fit for you and offers all that you want from your time there. It is also a good idea to visit the CSD department during your campus visit. When you are researching the institution, search the department Web site for the department phone number. Then call and ask to speak to an undergraduate advisor or his or her secretary. Make an appointment on the day of your visit to discuss the program. Explain that you are a high school student.

During the appointment, ask the advisor:

- What are the prerequisites to entering the program?
- Is there an application process to enter the undergraduate major? If so, what courses are required? May I have the application?
- What is the average GPA?
- Do you have a list of courses that are offered for undergraduates?
- Is there an active NSSLHA chapter? What types of activities does the chapter do?
- Is there a graduate program for audiology and/or speech-language pathology?
- What percentage of your students who apply for graduate school in audiology or speech-language pathology get into a program?

# Order a Complimentary Subscription to NSSLHA's Newsletter

It is not too soon to start learning about the academic and professional issues CSD majors face. The NSSLHA newsletter, *News & Notes*, is an excellent resource to find out more about what is going on with CSD students, CSD programs, and the professions. Email NSSLHA at nsslha@asha.org and let them know you are a high school student who would like a complimentary subscription to *News & Notes*.

## Get Involved

By getting involved in clubs, groups, or teams, you will learn more about yourself and other people, and be more knowledgeable about a variety of topics. Getting involved can help you develop good interpersonal skills and self-confidence that will be important for success in CSD. Depending on your interests and what is available at your high school or in your community, you may want to consider getting involved with the student newspaper, drama club, band, yearbook, prayer group, student council, track team, or other team sports. Beside being a great way to meet people and enjoy great experiences, colleges usually like students to be well-rounded. Plus, having a variety of experiences may make it easier to relate to your clients and their families. Clients usually brighten up when clinicians have experience with an activity that they currently, or used to, do. If you decide one day to work with children, having many different experiences of your own to draw upon could be very helpful in putting them at ease and making them feel comfortable with you.

## Consider Working Part-Time

Working while in high school may or may not be the best option for you. Count how many hours of homework you have each night, average sleep that you need to feel alert, and the time you devote for extracurricular activities, such as band, cross-country practice, speech club, drama, etc. Also consider if you have easy access to transportation (e.g., car or bike). Speak with your parents/guardians about how they feel about you working. If you decide to work, find a part-time job that will give you experience related to CSD. Apply to be a day-camp counselor for children with special needs, child care worker, nursing home worker, or tutor. Any experience you gain can be useful down the road either in helping you understand material in your classes, even applying to graduate school, and working with clients.

## Volunteer

Consider volunteering at a hospital if the medical setting interests you. Volunteering at a hospital is a great way to learn about the medical professions. You can request to volunteer in the hearing; ear, nose, and throat; or speech-language pathology clinics. Volunteering in the emergency room, admitting, birthing floor, and other areas of the hospital will give you a great insight on how a hospital functions. You will draw on these experiences when you are taking undergraduate and graduate courses in CSD. It can also be an excellent way to start thinking about any work settings you may one day consider.

## CONCLUSION

High school students seem to be getting busier and busier all the time. With schoolwork, extracurriculars, part-time jobs, spending time with friends, and the stress of applying to college, it may feel like you do not have any time left to spend planning for a career that seems so far off. Reading through this list, though, should help you see that there are many things you can start doing now that will have a positive impact down the road. Some of these suggestions, such as taking science and writing classes, are good ideas regardless of what major you decide to pursue. Other suggestions, such as job shadowing may require a little more effort, but learning early on that you are interested in pursuing a particular degree can give you the advantage in a sometimes competitive college application process. On the other hand, learning early about what you really *do not* want to do for a living can save you a lot of hassle later on (such as finding yourself behind in credits once you change majors, or needing to change colleges because the path you thought you wanted to pursue turns out to be not for you). For many people, deciding on a major and/or career is something that takes time.

# CHAPTER 7

# Advice for Freshman Year

## INTRODUCTION

As a freshman in college, you will likely be taking university-wide courses that are required for graduation (e.g., biology, writing, calculus, anthropology, etc.). Many freshmen find their first year is spent fulfilling the general education course requirements, and there are limited choices for coursework in a CSD major. Sometimes it can be confusing knowing what you need to take when it comes time to choose classes. Fortunately, every student has an academic advisor. Get to know your academic advisor because he or she will help you navigate through the required courses and can offer advice on selecting any electives toward your major (if that is an option during your freshman year). This chapter provides advice for achieving success throughout your freshman year and Figure 7-1 can be used as a checklist to keep track of your progress.

## Join Your Campus Chapter of NSSLHA

As a freshman, you may find there are a number of organizations, groups, and clubs that are eager for your involvement. Consider joining your local NSSLHA chapter. Ask your academic advisor to put you in contact with the chapter president. Being involved with NSSLHA will give you opportunities to be friends with the people who are in your major as well as get involved with the issues that concern your local chapter. However, do not be surprised if you are one of the only freshmen there. You are already ahead of the game by knowing what you want to do! Take this time to learn from more experienced students who can give you advice about your current and future classes. Refer back to Chapter 3 for detailed information on what NSSLHA is and what it does.

## Join NSSLHA

In addition to your local NSSLHA chapter, you may want to join the national organization. For more information about the benefits of joining NSSLHA, read Chapter 3 or visit the NSSLHA Web site at http://www.nsslha.org and click on the "Join" link.

☐ Join your campus chapter of NSSLHA.

☐ Join NSSLHA.

☐ Make a timeline of your courses from now until graduation.

☐ Study smart.

☐ Take a time management course.

☐ Take a study skills class.

☐ Learn APA.

☐ Make your face and name known.

☐ Take advantage of professors' office hours.

☐ Communicate with your NSSLHA Regional Councilor.

☐ Find out if your university has an Undergraduate Research Program.

☐ Observe speech and/or hearing therapy at your campus's CSD clinic.

☐ Observe an audiologist or SLP outside of your university.

☐ Save your textbooks and notes.

☐ Find out if you have to apply to your undergraduate major.

☐ Create a resumé.

☐ Download a graduate school application.

☐ Keep a college contact list.

☐ Volunteer at a clinic or hospital.

☐ Apply for a summer job related to CSD.

**Figure 7-1** Checklist for freshman year

## Make a Timeline of Your Courses from Now until Graduation

You may be feeling a little overwhelmed with all the courses you need to take before you graduate. Keep yourself organized by making a timeline of all your courses from your first year through graduation. To make sure you have the right course information, make an appointment with your academic advisor to plan out your coursework. The outline will ensure that you avoid taking unnecessary courses, and can help you target elective courses that you are interested in taking. Your advisor will assist you in ensuring you enroll in courses according to when the courses are offered. For example, some courses are offered in the fall of every other year. If you are unaware of when courses are offered and you neglect to take them when they are offered, your graduation could be delayed. With a timeline, you can avoid this type of problem.

Some students like to take all of their university-wide requirements first; others like to take university-wide requirements concurrently with prerequisites and requirements for their major. Mixing up challenging and easy courses can help you maintain a healthy and manageable academic course load. However, you may not be able to choose when you take some courses, depending upon your university and availability of courses.

## Study Smart

With all the exciting things that go on during the first year in college, some freshman have a hard time keeping focused on studying. Remember that your grades will be evaluated when you apply for graduate school and scholarships. To enter most graduate schools, you need a minimum of a 3.0 grade point average (GPA) on a 4.0 scale. However, the most competitive schools accept students who have at least a 3.5 GPA. What if, like many students, your GPA is not where you need it to be? A rocky first semester does not mean you lost your chance at getting into graduate school. Many students go through an adjustment period when they first get to college, and sometimes grades are not as high as a student would like. If your grades are lower than you want or need them to be, most campuses have a number of resources available to help you achieve academic success. There may be writing centers and tutors who can help you, as well as professor office hours. If you know you want to go on to get a graduate degree in audiology or speech-language pathology or a doctorate in audiology, use these resources to their fullest potential.

## Take a Time Management Course

The move from high school, where homework is done and turned in on a regular basis, to college, where the grade for an entire course may rest on a handful of papers or tests, can be challenging. Many students find that suddenly they are overwhelmed by papers and midterms due all at the same time. Taking a time management course early in your college career can help you effectively keep on top of your assignments and get the most out of each of your classes. Most schools offer these courses to freshmen. Sometimes they are called "Introduction to College Life," and usually teach time management skills, which will allow you to balance your time for courses, study, work, spirituality, volunteerism, and social life. These are lifelong skills, as you will need to balance multiple aspects of your life long after you graduate (e.g., being a professor/researcher/clinician, being a spouse, being a parent, focusing on your spirituality, volunteering, earning continuing education units to maintain certification, and building/maintaining relationships with family and friends). Fortunately, these are all aspects that you can balance when you learn good time management skills.

# Take a Study Skills Class

Study skills may or may not be incorporated into an "Introduction to College Life" course. Most of the skills you need to make good grades in college are different from the skills used in high school (e.g., the notes you take and textbooks you read are higher in quality and quantity). Courses on study skills usually advertise that they will teach you "how to study smarter without studying harder." If you are not required to take an introductory course that teaches study skills, but are interested in making the most of your study time, contact your academic advisor to see what resources your school offers.

# Learn APA

Many freshman English classes want students to use the Modern Language Association (MLA) style when writing papers. However, in the field of CSD, American Psychological Association (APA) documentation is used when writing papers. If you are given a choice to use MLA or APA style of documentation, practice using APA. Purchase a book from a local bookstore or go to the APA Web site (http://www.apa.org) to learn how to properly format and document references in papers and reports.

# Make Your Face and Name Known

Make yourself seen around the department and let professors get to know you. This allows them to see you as a freshman and watch you grow throughout your college career. When you have a class with these professors, you will probably feel more comfortable approaching them with questions. Also, when applying for graduate school, these professors will be able to write you powerful letters of recommendation. *Don't be just a number!*

# Take Advantage of Professors' Office Hours

Who better to help you with questions or problems than the professor teaching the class? Meet with your professors during their office hours if you do not understand something or want to learn more about a topic. Do not be afraid to email your professor, stay after class, and seek help if you need it. Professors are being paid to teach you the concepts and answer your questions. Get your money's worth. Most professors enjoy students who are inquisitive and want to learn. By regularly making use of office hours, you may find you connect really well with a particular professor. This kind of relationship can be helpful if you decide to apply to graduate school and need recommendations or even a faculty mentor.

# Communicate with Your
# NSSLHA Regional Councilor

Your NSSLHA Regional Councilor from the NSSLHA Executive Council, who also is a student, is a great resource. You can find out which Regional Councilor is assigned to your state by visiting the Council page of the NSSLHA Web site located at http://www.nsslha.org. Ask any questions that you have about being a student and future professional in CSD. Your NSSLHA Regional Councilor may have access to information that is not readily available on your campus.

# Find Out If Your University Has
# an Undergraduate Research Program

Research programs teach research procedures and pair students with a researcher in their area of interest. This is an excellent way to learn how research is conducted and to become knowledgeable about a specific topic. Contact your CSD department chairperson or a CSD professor to find out if this opportunity is available to you. If your college does not have a specific program (usually only larger universities have them), contact the head of your department and ask if you can assist a professor in the department with research. There may not be a program in place, but there may be professors in need of research assistance. At many universities, you can earn academic credit by registering the experience as an independent study.

# Observe Speech and/or Hearing
# Therapy at Your Campus's CSD Clinic

Observation at a campus communication sciences and disorders clinic is a great way to learn about clinical practice. As a freshman, any observations you do are separate from ASHA's required observation hours; these hours are simply a great way for you to learn more about the profession. You will learn more about these required hours during your junior or senior years. To observe, first find out if your campus has a CSD clinic, then contact the clinic director or coordinator. A clinic director is an audiologist or speech-language pathologist who is in charge of running a department's clinic. This is a great experience and a way to get to know the clinic director who may be a professor in your future courses. If there are opportunities to observe, make sure to ask about and follow any procedures required at the clinic, such as signing in, following a particular dress code, or how to interact with clients.

# Observe an Audiologist or SLP
# Outside of Your University

To learn more about professionals working outside an academic setting, you can observe an audiologist or SLP working in a hospital, school, or private practice. You can locate potential individuals to observe by looking through the phone book or speaking with professors or individuals associated with your campus clinic. Again, these hours are to help you learn more about the profession and are separate from ASHA's required observation hours. If possible, try to complete 10 to 15 hours of observations by the end of the school year. Observing now will help make the discussions in your future courses much more concrete (which may consequently make the material easier to learn). Come with questions for the audiologist or SLP.

## Save Your Textbooks and Notes

Students often look to the end of the semester as an opportunity to sell back books and make a little extra money. How disappointing it can be, though, when that text you originally paid $80.00 for, and sold back for $10.00, turns out to be a resource you wish you had for a graduate course. As you start taking courses that relate to your major, you will find it helpful to save your textbooks. Not only might they be required in another class, but they can be excellent resources and references for papers and projects (even in graduate school and professional practice). It is also a good idea to save your notes as references (e.g., psychology, education, and statistics notes).

Use 3-ring binders to organize your notes, with tabs to separate subjects. To make it easier to find your notes, write down all of the materials in the binder on two labels. Attach one sticky label to the spine of the binder, and the other to the front of the binder. The end of the semester is a good time to put your note binder together because the material is still fresh in your mind. Appendix A provides a complete list of items to help you get organized.

When you are in graduate school, you will be grateful that you have been organized since freshman year. To become a nationally-certified clinician after graduate school, you will be required to take a comprehensive exam that covers all of the material from your undergraduate major and graduate coursework. It will make preparation for this exam a lot less stressful if you have that binder for reference. Furthermore, these textbooks and notes are the foundation of your professional library.

## Find Out If You Have to Apply to Your Undergraduate Major

Some schools require students to apply separately for acceptance into their undergraduate major. Talk with your academic advisor about this early. Sometimes students have to submit their transcript, letters of recommendation, resumé, and statement of purpose for going into the profession to the department to be considered for the major. This process is similar to applying to graduate school. However, other programs admit any student who has been admitted into the university without an additional application process.

# Create a Resumé

A resumé is a one-page document that tells a prospective employer about your professional experience, education, and interests. While you may not have much professional experience yet, it is a good idea to keep track of all the different jobs and positions you hold. Record all of your work experiences, volunteer services, and educational experiences in a working resumé. Final resumés generally follow specific formats. If your campus has a career center, you can make an appointment to learn how to write a resumé. If your campus does not have a career center, ask a librarian to help you find a book about writing resumés. Starting a resumé now will help you realize what you need to accomplish over the next few years. Furthermore, a resumé will be useful when you are applying to honor societies, undergraduate programs (if applicable), honor societies, graduate programs, jobs, and scholarships. Refer to Chapter 28 for more information on drafting a resumé.

# Download a Graduate School Application

If graduate school is a possibility, begin now looking at graduate school applications in preparation for what you will need to do when you are ready to apply. Go online and download an application form from a dream school or CSD program that you would like to attend. Look over the application now, and you can spend the next few years making sure that you have enough experiences to fill in the application as an ideal candidate. Before you know it, your "dream school" may become a reality.

# Keep a College Contact List

The college contact worksheet in Figure 7-2 is an excellent resource for keeping track of important names, numbers, and addresses. Update this list every academic school year, and it will be a cinch to contact key individuals when you have questions. This list will also make it easier when you fill out scholarship and graduate school applications.

# Volunteer at a Clinic or Hospital

Keeping yourself actively involved in the profession is key—not to mention that graduate schools look at community service. The summer break is an ideal time to gain experience in a clinic or hospital that treats communication disorders. If you do not know where to look for these opportunities, ask your NSSLHA advisor, academic program director, or visit the ASHA On-line Career Center at http://www.asha.org for a list of professionals in your area. Building good relationships with a clinic or hospital now may mean future volunteer opportunities, or even employment opportunities down the line. Keep track of your volunteer experiences on your resumé.

This form can be updated every academic school year to assist you when visiting programs, completing grants and scholarship applications, completing college applications, or just to keep track of people in the profession with whom you come in contact.

**Name of University Academic Advisor:** _____

Address: _____

Phone Number: _____

Email: _____

**Name of CSD Academic Advisor:** _____

Address: _____

Phone Number: _____

Email: _____

**Name of NSSLHA Advisor:** _____

Address: _____

Phone Number: _____

Email: _____

**Name of NSSLHA Chapter President:** _____

Address: _____

Phone Number: _____

Email: _____

**Name of NSSLHA Regional Councilor:** _____

Address: _____

Phone Number: _____

Email: _____

*(continues)*

**Figure 7-2** College contact worksheet

Page 2

**Name of Mentor:** _____

Address: _____

Phone Number: _____

Email: _____

**Name of Professor Who Can Write You a Letter of Recommendation:** _____

Address: _____

Phone Number: _____

Email: _____

**Name of State Association:** _____

Phone Number: _____

Web Site: _____

Email: _____

**Other:** _____

Phone Number: _____

Web Site: _____

Email: _____

**Other:** _____

Phone Number: _____

Web Site: _____

Email: _____

**Figure 7-2** (Continued)

## Apply for a Summer Job Related to CSD

If you are like most students, you need to spend your summer making money for the upcoming school year. Instead of working at a fast food restaurant or in the mall, work at a day camp for children with disabilities or become a respite worker. (Respite workers provide care to an individual with a disability, allowing parents or caregivers to have time to run errands or have some much-needed personal time to themselves.) Working with children and adults with disabilities is a fantastic way to build experiences that will help you in your professional career.

Do a Web search or look in your local phone book to find respite services that may be in need of employees. Search the ASHA Web site to find camps for children with special needs. Go to http://www.asha.org for more information. Start researching for a summer job two or three months in advance. The pay is usually better than fast food or other seasonal work, looks great on a resumé, and will give you experiences that will make some of the material you learn in your major more salient.

## CONCLUSION

As a freshman, many new experiences and learning opportunities are open to you. Enjoy this time, but also stay focused on your long-term goal: to work as a CSD professional. While your career as a practicing audiologist, speech-language pathologist, or speech-language-hearing scientist may be a long way off, by using the suggestions in this chapter you can gain valuable experiences that will follow you through your education into your professional career.

# CHAPTER 8

# Advice for Sophomore Year

## INTRODUCTION

As a sophomore, you are likely to take at least a few courses in or related to your major. For example, you may be taking an Introduction to CSD and Introduction to Linguistics course. This can be very exciting, as you are beginning to really learn the concepts that form the foundation of professional work. As you continue through your studies, make sure you make time for yourself. Students in CSD tend to overwork themselves. If you find yourself doing this, try doing something fun with friends at least once a week. Relaxation and laughter are good for you—so is achieving balance between your academic, social, and personal commitments. When you take time for yourself, you will probably feel more refreshed and ready to tackle your homework and readings. Use the checklist in Figure 8-1 to identify things you can do to make your sophomore year as successful as possible.

## Renew Your Local Chapter Membership

If you joined your local chapter of NSSLHA, renew your membership. If you did not join as a freshman, then get involved this year. Keep track of what activities the chapter is holding and participate in the events that interest you. Also, get to know your Chapter President and Chapter Advisor. Record the events that you participate in on your resumé.

## Renew Your NSSLHA Membership

If you joined the national organization as a freshman, be sure to renew your membership. If you did not, now is your chance. Visit the NSSLHA Web site at http://www.nsslha.org on occasion. The site will keep you up to date on educational opportunities, conventions, student scholarships, and more.

## Volunteer for a Committee or Run for an Office in Your Local Chapter of NSSLHA

Building relationships and staying involved in your department is the best way to gain access to resources that will help you throughout your academic career. Stay connected to your local chapter and its events by being involved. Joining

- [ ] Renew your local chapter membership.
- [ ] Renew your NSSLHA membership.
- [ ] Volunteer for a committee or run for an office in your local chapter of NSSLHA.
- [ ] Apply for student membersip in your state's Speech-Language-Hearing Association.
- [ ] Volunteer at a state association convention.
- [ ] Focus on your GPA.
- [ ] Start exploring a specific discipline or professional area of interest.
- [ ] Consider taking a foreign language or sign language class.
- [ ] Consider taking a class on cultural diversity.
- [ ] Consider getting a minor.
- [ ] Speak with a graduate student in the CSD program.
- [ ] Revise your resumé.
- [ ] Get to know your professors and/or maintain existing relationships.
- [ ] Apply to volunteer at the ASHA Convention.
- [ ] Find a summer job and/or volunteer at places related to CSD.
- [ ] Take care of any teaching certification requirements as an undergraduate.

**Figure 8-1** Checklist for sophomore year

a committee to solve a problem, planning an event, or achieving a goal can be a great way to network and have fun. Consider running for an office in your local NSSLHA chapter, where you can gain leadership experience that will be important to graduate schools and of interest to future employers.

## Apply for Student Membership in Your State's Speech-Language-Hearing Association

Most state Speech-Language-Hearing Associations allow students to become members for a reduced fee. Applications may ask for a signature from the head of your department to verify that you are a student. Most state associations have a Web site where you can download an application. You can locate the state association in your area in the student resources section of the NSSLHA Web site at http://www.nsslha.org. State associations usually have newsletters and conferences to provide information beyond what is taught in the classroom.

## Volunteer at a State Association Convention

If you are interested in new volunteer experiences, consider volunteering at a state speech, language, and hearing association convention. State associations are always looking for volunteers to help at registration desks, stuffing envelopes, and taking care of paperwork. Most conventions are during the first half of the calendar year, but planning for these meetings is a huge undertaking and your help may be needed at other times in the year. Call your state association to ask whom to contact to volunteer at the convention. When you are not volunteering at the convention, you can attend educational sessions. Remember to add the volunteer experience and your educational sessions to your resumé.

## Focus on Your GPA

Being a strong candidate to a graduate program means having a solid GPA. A minimum 3.0 is required for many graduate programs, but many of the more competitive schools prefer students with at least a 3.5. If your grades are not where you would like them to be, meet with your academic advisor to consider ways you can improve. Make use of the resources at your disposal, including professors, classmates, tutoring labs, and writing centers to get the support you need to achieve your academic goals. Also realize that in your graduate school application, you can explain that your grades were lower during certain semesters, but you have been a strong student since then. (Many schools have applicants report an overall GPA and a GPA for the major.)

## Start Exploring a Specific Discipline or Professional Area of Interest

It is never too early to start planning for your future. Use this time to start asking more questions about what really interests you in CSD and start finding educational and volunteer opportunities in that area of interest. Let your program's faculty and the resources available from national and local NSSLHA assist you in identifying your interests.

NSSLHA members can join ASHA's Special Interest Divisions for a reduced fee. Special Interest Divisions are specialty groups that focus on a particular area of the profession. Every division publishes a newsletter for its members. There are 16 divisions currently recognized by ASHA. To learn more about these divisions visit http://www.asha.org.

To help you choose electives, do your research on the graduate school that you may consider and try to select courses that will improve your chances of being accepted into that program. Visit the Web site of the graduate level CSD program you are interested in to see what courses are required for undergraduates that are not required in your program. If your program offers these courses, take them. If your program does not offer the needed courses, look to see if another university offers them online. Contact a potential graduate program and see if the credit would transfer. It is never too early to start preparing for graduate school. Use your undergraduate time wisely.

## Consider Taking a Foreign Language or Sign Language Class

Employers often prefer to hire job candidates who know some Spanish, sign language, or other foreign languages. The profession is in great need of more bilingual clinicians. You will be very marketable when you graduate if you know a foreign language. No matter what setting you work in as a professional, you will be grateful to have more than one way to communicate with others.

## Consider Taking a Class on Cultural Diversity

As a CSD professional, you will come in contact with many different people from a wide range of cultural, ethnic, and religious backgrounds. To help you deal appropriately and effectively with these clients and their families, consider taking a class on cultural diversity. Many CSD departments offer these courses. However, taking a course on cultural diversity through another department will also prove to be very valuable.

## Consider Getting a Minor

Some students have a minor, but it is not a requirement in the field. Sometimes, there is not enough time or financial means to earn a minor and graduate in four years. However, if there is an area of interest that you would like to pursue, then go for it! Sign Language, Psychology, Special Education, Elementary Education, Family Studies, Statistics, Linguistics, Gerontology, Communications, and Spanish are some common minors that students in CSD programs consider.

## Speak with a Graduate Student in the CSD Program

Graduate students can be very knowledgeable and may be more approachable than some professors. They can let you know what to expect after graduating with your bachelors degree. If your school only has an undergraduate program, contact your NSSLHA Regional Councilor (RC) to find a graduate student in your region who can answer your questions and give advice. You can find out how to contact your RC by going to the Executive Council section of the NSSLHA Web site at http://www.nsslha.org.

# Revise Your Resumé

By now you probably have a number of volunteer and work experiences that are related to CSD. It is a good idea to include all of these great experiences on your resumé (you will be surprised how quickly you can forget important information). Most campuses have a career center that can help students write a resumé. Make an appointment at your career center and bring your most recent resumé for feedback on improvements. The resumé will be helpful when you are applying for summer jobs, completing graduate school applications, applying to honor societies, and filling out scholarship forms.

# Get to Know Your Professors and/or Maintain Existing Relationships

This was excellent advice for freshman, but it becomes even more important for sophomores. Now that you are further along in your studies and the material is getting more complicated, your professors can help when you are confused about assignments or materials. They can also act as mentors to help you identify specific interests and provide suggestions for achieving your academic and career goals. Utilize their office hours—that's why they have them.

# Apply to Volunteer at the ASHA Convention

The ASHA convention, held each November, is a great place for CSD students to volunteer. Currently, students who are accepted as volunteers receive a full refund equivalent to the early-bird registration fee after completing eight to ten hours of volunteer service. Student volunteer applications are usually announced in April and the deadline for applications is June. Information on the student volunteer application, as well as the volunteer program, is available on the NSSLHA and ASHA Web sites.

# Find a Summer Job and/or Volunteer at Places Related to CSD

Consider volunteering at a hospital or clinic during the summer after your sophomore year to gain more experience working with individuals with communication disorders and the professionals who assess, diagnose, and treat them. Or look for a job working as a counselor at a day camp for children with disabilities or as a respite worker who assists individuals with disabilities and their families. Consider saving some of your money to cover your registration fees and expenses to attend the ASHA Convention or state association convention next year.

## Take Care of Any Teaching Certification Requirements as an Undergraduate

If you think you might be interested in working in a school setting, make sure you know the requirements. In fact, a state may require you to have a teaching certificate to work in a hospital because you could work with children from schools that do not have an audiologist on staff or have an SLP shortage. Most states require professionals to take certain special education coursework and have teaching experience. To learn more about teaching certification requirements, contact your academic advisor, NSSLHA chapter advisor, state board of education, and/or an audiologist or SLP who works in a school.

Regardless of whether or not you work in the schools, education classes will be beneficial. These classes will strengthen your teaching skills. You will also have the opportunity to interact with other future professionals, such as special education teachers, general education teachers, occupational therapists, physical therapists, and more. Collaborating with others is an important skill to learn because it can be beneficial to working on interdisciplinary teams for the benefit of your future clients.

### CONCLUSION

By the sophomore year, students are getting deeper into their CSD coursework and closer to working with individuals with speech, language, hearing and swallowing disorders. This chapter provides some ways beyond your regular coursework to become even more involved in your future profession. Refer back to the checklist (Figure 8-1) at the beginning of the chapter and use it to help you further advance on your path to becoming an audiologist, speech-language pathologist, or speech and hearing scientist.

# CHAPTER 9

## Advice for Junior Year

### INTRODUCTION

Junior year is likely the first year when most of your classes will be in CSD. You have probably completed most of your university-wide courses, and now can focus on the area that interests you most—your major! At this point, you are one year away from applying to a graduate program in CSD. If you are going into audiology, you should start considering whether to pursue a Doctorate of Audiology (see Chapter 21) or a Doctorate of Philosophy (see Chapter 22). If you are going into speech-language pathology, start considering if you want to pursue a master's (see Chapter 18) or continue your study toward a Doctorate of Philosophy degree (see Chapter 23). You should continue to build your resumé with experiences that will make you an ideal candidate for a graduate program. This chapter provides tips to help you survive your junior year, and the checklist in Figure 9-1 can be used to keep track of your progress.

### Start Researching CSD Graduate Programs

By now you should have an idea of whether you want to pursue a graduate degree. This is a good time to start researching graduate programs that are of interest to you. You might start your research at the Graduate School Fair hosted by NSSLHA during the ASHA convention. Here, students can gather information about the different graduate programs available and can meet with faculty from many of the schools. As you are considering different programs, remember that to become an ASHA-certified audiologist or SLP you must complete graduate coursework from a program accredited by the Council on Academic Accreditation in Audiology and Speech-Language Pathology (CAA) of the American Speech-Language-Hearing Association (ASHA). A list of these programs is available through the online graduate guide of accredited programs listed in the Student section of the ASHA Web site (http://www.asha.org). Utilize these resources to search for graduate opportunities in the professions. As you begin looking, keep an open mind. Look at many different schools across the country—the right program for you and your academic interests could be across the street or across the country, but you will never know if you do not thoroughly investigate your options.

- [ ] Start researching CSD graduate programs.
- [ ] Attend and volunteer at the ASHA Convention in November.
- [ ] Attend and volunteer at your state association convention (again).
- [ ] Apply for a regional councilor position in NSSLHA.
- [ ] Remain focused on your GPA.
- [ ] Update your resumé.
- [ ] Start researching financial aid options to fund your graduate studies.
- [ ] Find out if you can participate in a directed study during your senior year.
- [ ] Begin preparation for the Graduate Record Exam.

**Figure 9-1** Checklist for junior year

## Attend and Volunteer at the ASHA Convention in November

The further along you get in your studies, the more you will get out of attending the ASHA convention. If you cannot afford to attend, consider applying to volunteer. See Chapter 30 for more information on the convention.

## Attend and Volunteer at Your State Association Convention (Again)

While the national ASHA convention is a fantastic place to attend sessions and be exposed to hot topics of interest in the profession, your state convention offers informative sessions, access to vendors and resources, is less expensive, and is usually closer than the national convention. Presenters and sessions are always changing, so if you have attended the state convention in the past, be sure to attend again. Now that you have taken multiple courses in your program, the sessions will reinforce what you have been learning. If you have not previously attended, commit to going during your junior year. This is an excellent way of networking with students and professionals and will help you begin connecting with the professional community.

## Apply for a Regional Councilor (RC) Position in NSSLHA

Getting involved at the national level of NSSLHA will give you the opportunity to meet future CSD leaders, as well as make contact with leaders of ASHA.

A Regional Councilor (RC) acts as a liaison between the NSSLHA Executive Council and the chapters within the region. The RC regularly communicates with NSSLHA chapters, attends biannual Executive Council meetings, and sits on an ASHA board or committee. Applications for Regional Councilor are usually accepted every February and are available on the NSSLHA Web site. To learn more about the position, contact the RC for your region by going to the council page on the NSSLHA Web site.

## Remain Focused on Your GPA

As you move from the general and introductory courses into more specialized topics in your major, you may find the material is more interesting, but it may also be more challenging. With the decision to apply to graduate school around the corner, it is more important than ever to maintain your GPA to make yourself a competitive candidate. As mentioned in earlier chapters, most graduate schools require a minimum of 3.0 GPA, with some requiring a minimum 3.5 GPA. If you find you need help, make use of the resources available on campus, find a graduate student who can tutor you, or work with your professors during their office hours.

## Update Your Resumé

If you have been following the advice for freshman (Chapter 7) and sophomores (Chapter 8), you should have started your resumé. Read Chapter 28, Resumé and Interview Preparation, for more information on updating resumés. If you have not created one, now is the time to get started.

## Start Researching Financial Aid Options to Fund Your Graduate Studies

While graduate school can be a considerable financial commitment, there are a number of great options for helping fund this stage in your education. Graduate assistantships, loans, and grants are often available, depending on the university you plan to attend and your particular situation. Refer to Chapter 4 for more information about financing your graduate education.

## Find Out If You Can Participate in a Directed Study During Your Senior Year

A directed study is an opportunity for a student to work on a research project with a professor, based on a common research interest. You may work along side that professor for a semester, in a clinic or lab, while earning academic credit. If your program does not already have a directed study environment in place, introduce the concept to them. This is a great way to get your research career started with a mentor who you trust to guide you through the process.

This experience may be useful when applying for research-related positions as a graduate student; professors usually like to hire students who have research experience.

## Begin Preparation for the Graduate Record Exam (GRE)

The Graduate Record Exam (GRE) is the entrance examination required for most graduate-level programs. These scores are often used to nominate students for fellowships, which can pay a student's tuition and provide a stipend. The three sections on the GRE are written analytical, verbal, and quantitative. The written analytical section is based on a 6-point grading scale. The verbal and quantitative sections are worth up to 800 points each. The average GRE acceptance score for a graduate CSD program is probably higher than the overall university required score. Find out what range of scores you need to be accepted into your desired graduate program.

Visit the GRE Web site at http://www.gre.org for registration information. Create a study plan that works best for you. You may want to purchase a review book with a CD-ROM to help direct your studying and to take practice tests. To save money, find out if a library on your campus has GRE review books.

Another way to prepare for the GRE is with a review course. Your university may offer GRE review courses or recommend a company that provides this service. However, you should realize that these courses can cost from $400 to $2,000. Plan accordingly if you choose to take a review course. Instead of a formal course, some review agencies offer online courses that are in the $100 to $300 range. Check with review agencies for exact prices. Before committing a significant amount of money to a review course, take a practice exam in a GRE review book to get a sense of how much preparation you may need.

## CONCLUSION

Junior year is when many students really hit their stride—they are comfortable in their college environment, understand what is expected of them, and know what to expect from their courses. It is also an exciting time for CSD majors because they are taking more advanced classes. While it may feel like graduation is still a long way off, the application process for attending graduate school is just around the corner. Junior year is the perfect time to start investigating graduate programs and preparing for the GRE. Use the checklist at the beginning of this chapter to keep track of what you need to accomplish to prepare for what may be a busy year.

# CHAPTER 10

# Advice for Senior Year

## INTRODUCTION

At last! Senior year! You have accomplished a great deal during your CSD studies and should be proud of all your hard work. You are now faced with some important decisions about what direction to take after graduation. Besides all these important decisions (where to apply to graduate school, how to pay for more education), you still have a rigorous year of coursework ahead. Senior year can be very demanding. Your academic courses will become more in-depth and your homework and projects may become more involved. Plus, you will spend much of the fall and early winter preparing your graduate school applications. This chapter provides tips on making the most of this busy year, and the checklist in Figure 10-1 can be used to keep track of your progress.

## Take the GRE Early in the Fall

Do not wait until the last minute to take the GRE. Sign up for the early fall examination. This way, if you need to raise your scores, you have time to retake the exam before application deadlines arrive. Plus, if you do well the first time, then you will not need to worry about the GRE ever again. However, if you have to take the exam more than once, it is perfectly okay. Many students aspire to have high scores on the GRE and retest several times.

Consider taking a review course for the GRE if you are dissatisfied with your scores. Some universities offer review courses for sections of the GRE (e.g., verbal section) for a small fee. Ask your academic advisor or office of student affairs if any GRE courses are being offered at your university. Inquire about review courses through a learning center or a professional test-taking service in your area. Ask if an online course is offered so that you can work at your own pace. Keep in mind that some of the courses through testing centers can be quite costly. An on-line course may cost $100, but a review course or private tutor could cost $2,000 or more.

Make sure you know the scores that you will need for acceptance into the programs you are interested in and what scores are needed to be competitive for fellowships (which often require high GRE scores). If your scores are at or above the minimum scores to get into a program and your other areas

☐  Take the GRE early in the fall.

☐  Apply for graduate school in late fall or early winter.

☐  Apply for financial aid and other scholarship programs in late fall or early winter.

☐  Keep track of all deadlines for applications.

☐  Apply to graduate programs that share your interests.

☐  If accepted to several graduate programs, decide which you want to attend.

☐  Determine how much money you will need for graduate school.

☐  Ask about an assistantship position.

☐  Find out if your graduate program begins in the summer.

☐  Decide if you want to write a thesis.

☐  Attend the ASHA Convention in November.

☐  Volunteer at the ASHA convention if you have not already done so.

☐  Consider all your options.

**Figure 10-1**  Checklist for senior year

of application are strong (e.g. GPA, letters of recommendation, volunteer experience, and essays), then you may not need to pay thousands of dollars to get superior GRE scores. Speak with the academic program's department chair or advisor where you are applying to see how much GRE scores are emphasized when reviewing applications.

## Apply for Graduate School in Late Fall or Early Winter

Even if applications are not due until February or later, get your application materials together and mailed in early. Ask faculty members in your department, who know your skills and work ethic, to write positive letters of recommendation, and give them time to write the letters so that they will not be rushed. Give the professors a copy of your resumé, the letter of recommendation form, information on the deadline for submission, and a stamped envelope so they are not responsible for postage. Always follow up with a thank you note or card to let anyone who writes a recommendation know that you appreciate their time and effort.

Ask your NSSLHA advisor, or another faculty member, to review your graduate school application essays. If your school has a writing center that edits students' papers, make an appointment to review your essays. Since many programs do not have an interview process, your essays can be a powerful way to show how you are an ideal candidate for their program. Take the time to write your essays well.

## Apply for Financial Aid and Other Scholarship Programs in Late Fall or Early Winter

Refer to Chapter 4, Financing Your CSD Education, for more information on applying for financial aid and scholarships.

## Keep Track of All Deadlines for Applications

For fall admissions, some programs have deadlines as early as December 1. Make sure that you mail all of the information to the right departments well before the deadlines. After you mail your applications, you will need to call each university's CSD department to make sure they received all of the proper information. Sometimes letters of recommendation are lost or GRE scores are filed in the wrong place. Do not assume the departments received all of your information. Because most programs have many applicants, they will not contact you if they are missing part of your application. They simply will not review your application. Continue to call until you have verification that your application is complete. Use the Graduate School Application Worksheet in Figure 10-2 to help you keep track of your graduate school applications and the Graduate School Recommendation Sheet in Figure 10-3 to track letters of recommendation. As a reminder, be sure to send a thank you note to anyone who wrote a letter of recommendation for you.

## Apply to Graduate Programs That Share Your Interests

If you are really interested in research, make sure you apply to a program where professors are performing research that interests you. If you know you want to work in a school setting, choose a program with a strong focus on pediatric populations and school-based skills. Choosing a program that fits your interests increases the likelihood of finding professors who can act as mentors. If you want to focus on research, apply to a program with one or more professors who are researching in your area of interest and can help you in writing a thesis. Find out if the programs you are applying to offer research assistantships to first-year graduate students. Go to the department's Web site and read what each professor is currently researching.

This worksheet will help you organize your graduate school applications and stay on track of application requirements and deadlines.

**Name of Institution:**

Web Site for Program:

Web Site for Online Application:

Username for Online Application:

Password for Online Application:

Application Fee:

Address for Application Fee If Not Paid Online:

Address to Send Letters of Reference:

Address to Send Other Materials (and list specific materials):

Number of Letters of Reference Required:

Essay Prompt(s) and Page Length Requirements:

Due Date:

Date Sent:

Phone Number:

Other:

**Name of Institution:**

Web Site for Program:

Web Site for Online Application:

Username for Online Application:

Password for Online Application:

Application Fee:

Address for Application Fee If Not Paid Online:

Address to Send Letters of Reference:

Address to Send Other Materials (and list specific materials):

Number of Letters of Reference Required:

Essay Prompt(s) and Page Length Requirements:

Due Date:

Date Sent:

Phone Number:

Other:

*(continues)*

**Figure 10-2** Graduate school application worksheet

**Name of Institution:**

Web Site for Program:

Web Site for Online Application:

Username for Online Application:

Password for Online Application:

Application Fee:

Address for Application Fee If Not Paid Online:

Address to Send Letters of Reference:

Address to Send Other Materials (and list specific materials):

Number of Letters of Reference Required:

Essay Prompt(s) and Page Length Requirements:

Due Date:

Date Sent:

Phone Number:

Other:

**Name of Institution:**

Web Site for Program:

Web Site for Online Application:

Username for Online Application:

Password for Online Application:

Application Fee:

Address for Application Fee If Not Paid Online:

Address to Send Letters of Reference:

Address to Send Other Materials (and list specific materials):

Number of Letters of Reference Required:

Essay Prompt(s) and Page Length Requirements:

Due Date:

Date Sent:

Phone Number:

Other:

**Figure 10-2** (Continued)

Use this reference sheet when filling out graduate school applications to keep track of information for individuals who are writing your letters of reference.

**Professor:**

Title:

Address:

Phone:

Email:

Date Professor Prefers to Receive Packet:

Other:

**Professor:**

Title:

Address:

Phone:

Email:

Date Professor Prefers to Receive Packet:

Other:

**Professor:**

Title:

Address:

Phone:

Email:

Date Professor Prefers to Receive Packet:

Other:

**Former/Current Employer or Volunteer Coordinator (optional):**

Title:

Address:

Phone:

Email:

Date Employer/Volunteer Coordinator Prefers to Receive Packet:

Other:

**Figure 10-3** Graduate school recommendation sheet

# If Accepted to Several Graduate Programs, Decide Which You Want to Attend

If you have been accepted to several programs, you may have a very difficult decision before you. Ask yourself the following questions and weigh out what is most important:

- If finances were not an issue, what program would I prefer to attend?
- What program is the most affordable? What program is the most costly?
- Is the program near family or close friends? Will I know anyone at the university?
- Which cities have the highest and lowest costs of living?
- (If you have a family), how does my family feel about moving to a new city?
- Is the program offering me any scholarships or tuition waivers or are there scholarship possibilities after I am in the program for a year?
- Is there good public transportation?
- What is the city like? Is there a major city within a day's driving distance? (Being in or near a major city may be nice when you need to take a break from school because most major cities have recreational events throughout the year.)
- Is there a place of worship on or near campus that I would like to attend?
- Is there one or more professors with whom I would like to do research?
- Which programs have a good academic reputation?
- Do I want a program that is more research oriented or clinically oriented? Or do I like both aspects?
- When I called or emailed students in the graduate program, did they like the program? Did they seem overly stressed? Did they say that the professors are supportive and truly have an "open door" policy?
- Does the program require externships that are outside the city? (Some programs require a semester where you gain clinical experience in a town that is several hours away, in a rural area.)
- How long is the program? Master's programs can last two or three years. Doctoral programs can last from three to five years (the length may be variable).

Consider all these points and think about your long-term goals. Knowing yourself and what you want out of your graduate experience will help guide you through this decision.

# Determine How Much Money You Will Need for Graduate School

Once you have decided what school you will attend, create a budget for yourself. Also consider the cost of rent, bills (e.g., electric, water, heat, phone, cell phone, internet access, etc.), food, car payments, car insurance, books and new equipment (e.g., otoscope), furniture, clothing, and travel to visit family and friends. Plan how many hours you will work during graduate school. Talk to current graduate students and find out how many hours per week is realistically manageable.

Realize that not all graduate students work and you should take into account the stress involved in having a job. Some students work too many hours per week, and they miss out on learning much of the information they are paying to learn. Try to keep a healthy balance between school and what you may need to do to pay for school. At the end of your graduate program, you will need to pass the Praxis exam (a comprehensive exam that tests your knowledge in audiology or speech-language pathology). The exam is required for ASHA certification. If you end up working too much to cover the cost of your education and do not know the material covered on this examination, you may fail and be unable to practice. Ultimately, it is important to make time to learn the content because your knowledge base will affect the quality of services you provide to your clients and/or of your research. Keep all of this in mind as you are planning how to pay for your graduate education.

## Ask About an Assistantship Position

Research, teaching, clinical, and project assistantships are some of the assistantships available in graduate audiology and speech-language pathology programs. Some assistantships offer students a tuition waiver and/or stipend if they agree to assist a professor for a fixed number of hours per week (e.g., 15–20 hours). Most schools have a limited number of assistantships, so apply early and often. Assistantship opportunities may vary throughout the year. For instance, a professor may look for a research assistant after receiving a grant during the middle of an academic year. Contact a professor with whom you would like to work, let him or her know that you would be interested in an assistantship position, and stay in regular contact with that person if he or she indicates there may be something available later in the year.

## Find Out If Your Graduate Program Begins in the Summer

Some programs begin in the summer, others begin in the fall. This will be important since you will need to look for a place to live if you are moving to a new city.

## Decide If You Want to Write a Thesis

A thesis is a major project investigating a particular question. If you are interested in earning a doctorate, a thesis will help you decide if you enjoy the research process. Start thinking about research questions that you might want to address in your thesis.

# Attend the ASHA Convention in November

In Chapter 9, Advice for Junior Year, you were encouraged to attend the ASHA Convention. Now, in you senior year, it is even more important for you to have this experience. The many benefits of attending the ASHA Convention are discussed in Chapter 30, Going to the ASHA Convention.

# Volunteer at the ASHA Convention If You Have Not Already Done So

The good news is that students who volunteer at the convention get their registration paid. The bad news is that you can only be selected as a volunteer one time. If you applied last year and were accepted, you can not apply again. If you were not accepted, by all means, apply as a volunteer.

# Consider All Your Options

*Taking Time Off Before Entering a Graduate Program.* There are many reasons why a student may decide to take a year off before entering a graduate program, including a desire to travel, the need to work to save money, family obligations, or a feeling of being burned out and needing some time to recharge. Whatever your personal reasons for wanting to take time off, following are some tips for making this decision work smoothly with your plans for obtaining your graduate degree.

**Apply to Graduate Programs and (After Being Accepted) Ask If They Can Hold Your Place.** If you are early in your senior year and feel like you may need or want to take a year off before attending graduate school, keep in mind that a lot can change in a few months. Complete and submit your graduate school applications just as if you were planning on attending graduate school right after graduation. How you feel in November of your senior year could be very different than how you will feel in April—if you change your mind you can start school in the fall and will not be forced to wait a year. If you are accepted into a program and decide that you still want to take a year off, contact the department chair, and ask if your place can be held for one year. You may want to offer a reason why you would like to take a year off (e.g., to earn money to pay for school, to have a child, to establish in-state residency, to take a break, for medical reasons). It depends on the situation and the program whether they will be able to hold your place, but applying to programs knowing you can try to defer admission will give you more options than simply not applying.

**Get a Job That Utilizes Your CSD Skills and Knowledge.** If you are taking a year off to earn money to pay for your graduate education, look for a position that uses the knowledge and skills gained during your communication sciences and disorders coursework. If you are waiting to apply to graduate programs, the experience will be helpful to your application process. Likewise, having professional experience will make the material you learn in graduate school more salient once you enter your program. Consider the following settings as you are looking for job opportunities:

- Work in a hearing and speech center or hospital.
- Work as a teacher's aid at an elementary school.
- Be a substitute teacher. In some states, you may already have completed the education requirements. Contact the state's board of education for more information.

**You Are Taking Time Off Because You Are Unsure of What Professional Direction to Take.** If you are taking a year off because you are uncertain whether you want to go into audiology or speech-language pathology, consider taking a semester of classes in another major or observing a professional in the position that interests you. Sometimes, students in CSD become interested in a related field, such as medicine, nursing, psychology, social work, special education, physical therapy, occupational therapy, or music therapy. Take time to learn about your other interests. Graduate school in audiology or speech-language pathology will be easier if you are more confident about wanting a job after graduation.

**Study Abroad.** If you are taking a year off from school, take the opportunity to learn about other cultures. When you are an audiologist or SLP, you will interact with individuals from a variety of cultures. Studying abroad can assist you in having a better appreciation of different cultures and styles of communication. Furthermore, if you are interested in research, you may want to get ideas about research topics in CSD in relation to different cultures. If you go to a country that does not speak English, you can practice speaking the native language, a skill that may come in handy when you are on the job market. Plus, studying abroad is a fun experience!

**Consider Taking Courses for Teaching Certification If You Might Work in a School Setting.** If you think you may want to work in a school setting when you have obtained your graduate degree, you may need a teaching certificate to do this, depending on where you will be working. Begin preparing for this by taking education courses during your time off. Usually, the courses required for teaching certification are offered in the education department. Contact an advisor at your future graduate program to see what courses you will need to take. This will lighten your load when you are a graduate student.

### What If You Are Not Accepted to the Program You Want to Attend?

Many graduate programs in audiology and speech-language pathology are very competitive, and there is a chance that you may not be accepted at the school you most want to attend. Consider the following options if you are faced with this situation:

- Reapply for spring admissions. However, not all programs offer spring admissions. If the program does not have spring admissions, then reapply for fall admissions of the next year.

- Contact the department of your dream school and specifically ask what you can do to be more competitive. If possible, meet with someone from the department who reviews the applications. Ask him or her to review your application with you and find out how you can make your application stronger. Plan how you will accomplish the suggestions by the next application deadline.

- Find out if you can enroll in one or two graduate courses at your dream school even though you are not in the program. You may be able to register as a "special student." However, make sure that you study smart, perform well, and get an "A" in these classes. Then, the individuals who review your application next year will see that you have the potential to succeed in their program.

- If your GPA was not competitive, retake courses in which you earned a B or less. At some colleges, you can retake a few courses, but there is usually a limit. Often, this option is not advertised, so check your university's bulletin or make an appointment with your advisor. If you cannot retake courses, take courses related to CSD (e.g., education courses) to boost your GPA (make sure that you earn "As").

- If your GRE scores were not competitive, take a GRE review course.

- Earn a second major in another discipline. Consider Spanish, special education, business, or marketing.

- Take a year off to work in a position related to CSD.

- If your dream school is out of state, you may be eligible for in-state residency if you work for a year. However, contact the university to learn about all of the requirements for in-state residency. Check the university's Web site for phone numbers to call. Some programs try to maintain a ratio of in- and out-of-state students (usually with a higher percentage of in-state students).

## CONCLUSION

As you can see from this chapter, your senior year will be largely focused on what you will be doing after you graduate. Your studies should remain your primary focus, but on top of coursework, there is a lot to be done in preparation for your next step, whatever you choose it to be. Use this chapter for tips on successfully navigating the graduate school application process and to help guide your thinking as you plan for the next leg of your journey in communication sciences and disorders.

# CHAPTER 11

# Advice for Adults Returning to College to Pursue a CSD Degree

Sherri Webster, master's student, SLP, Western Washington University

## INTRODUCTION

After spending 15 years in TV production, I decided to return to college to pursue a second career in SLP. Since returning to college, I feel an amazing sense of accomplishment, partly because I'm more focused and disciplined than I was 20 years ago. Paying for my own education is another motivator. Now that I am paying for my education independently, it is more meaningful and valuable to me. I feel a greater sense of responsibility for doing well in my courses and learning the most from the instructors I am paying to teach me.

This chapter offers some tips that may help adults, like me, returning to college after taking time away from school get the most out of their CSD education. Figure 11-1 is a checklist of things to do to help ensure success.

## Know Your University's General University Requirements and Develop a Plan for Completing Them

About one-half of a bachelor's degree consists of General University Requirements (GURs) (or General Requirements, University Studies Program, or a number of other names). Primarily, GURs consist of courses in math, science, English, and writing. While many students complete these general course requirements at their 4-year college as part of their bachelor's degree studies, some adults returning to college may choose to complete GURs as part of an associate's degree from a community college or online degree program. Students sometimes choose to complete GURs at a community college because classes are less expensive and the community college environment can be smaller, geographically closer, or less intimidating than at a college or university. However, if you plan to take your GURs at a community college, make sure those credits will transfer to the college you plan to attend to obtain your CSD

- [ ] Know your university's General University Requirements and develop a plan for completing them.
- [ ] Be who you are.
- [ ] Take advantage of learning resources early in your academic career.
- [ ] Develop a study system that works for you.
- [ ] Learn while in class.
- [ ] Seek out resources for adults returning to college.
- [ ] Take things one day at a time.

**Figure 11-1** Checklist for adults returning to college

degree. Some colleges or universities may not recognize credits taken at a community college as fulfilling their credit requirements. (This can be due to many factors, so it is important to contact the CSD program's registrar's office to know how this effects you.) If your associate's degree GURs do not transfer to your bachelor's degree, you will need to retake the courses, which will cost more time and money.

## Be Who You Are

You may feel self-conscious when most students are younger than you. Remind yourself that you can learn something from everyone, regardless of age. Having more life experience puts you in the position to mentor younger students. Share your personal and professional experiences; you may have a lot to say that adds to the class discussion.

## Take Advantage of Learning Resources Early in Your Academic Career

Recognize that it is not a weakness to admit that you may need help learning how to learn. If you have been out of school for several years, you may have forgotten the study skills that many of your fellow students take for granted. Most colleges have learning centers to help you sharpen your study, reading, and comprehension skills. Many colleges have tutors for hire. All professors should have office hours where you can receive one-on-one help. Even the "A" students seek out tutors and learning centers to enhance their skills. Make use of all the resources available at your academic institution to help you learn and achieve your goals. Seek out additional resources as well, such as other chapters in this survival guide, that can help you become a successful student and professional.

## Develop a Study System That Works for You

You are responsible for your own study habits, and it takes time to develop systems that work best for you. Consider trying some of the following study skills. If you complete reading assignments prior to lectures you will feel more prepared, and you can contribute better to class discussions. Use a highlighter to pinpoint the key ideas in your reading assignments or write key ideas in the margins. If you are pressed for time, skim over the chapter before class and try to understand the main ideas. If your textbook has chapter objectives and summaries, pay close attention to this material, as it will help identify the key points from the reading. Make a study guide or flash cards for material discussed in class within 24 hours of the lecture. By putting things into your own words, you also take ownership of the material, which helps you retain it in your long-term memory. Experiment with different ways of taking and reviewing notes. As you learn more about yourself and what kind of learner you are, you will be able to create an effective, personal study system.

## Learn While in Class

It sounds like such simple advice, but some students "space out" during class while taking notes or listening to lectures. If you have other obligations outside of school, such as a spouse, children, or work, then you need to manage your time and focus carefully. Be an active learner during class. Constantly think how you will apply the material when you are a clinician or researcher. Ask and answer questions during class. If you need to, force yourself to learn by pretending that you will have a quiz at the end of class on the material that was taught.

## Seek Out Resources for Adults Returning to College

As an adult returning to college, you are not alone! There are resources available to help with a wide range of concerns that are particular to this special population of students. Visit Back to College (http://www.back2college.com) for a comprehensive list of resources, scholarships, and services for adults returning to college. Register for their bi-monthly electronic newsletter to access additional resources not listed on their Web site. If you are having difficulty managing your time, look into taking a time management course through your college or investigate time management resources at the library or a bookstore.

## Take Things One Day at a Time

At times, your CSD program may seem more challenging than anticipated. You may have a demanding job or family that needs you in addition to your coursework and observation. You may feel it is too much. However, most things in life that seem overwhelming are, in fact, achievable if you believe in yourself, stay focused, and take things one day at a time.

## CONCLUSION

For adults returning to college, the experience can be frightening, exhilarating, and challenging all at once. Some of the younger students sharing your classes may have the luxury of free time or freedom from other obligations, such as jobs or families, but may lack the experience you bring to discussions or the determination you have to achieve your academic and professional goals. To achieve success in your CSD studies, make use of the resources discussed in this chapter and seek out other returning adult students to create a support system for yourself.

# CHAPTER 12

# Advice for Students from Culturally and Linguistically Diverse Backgrounds

Vicki Deal-Williams, MS, ASHA Chief Staff Officer, Multicultural Concerns

## INTRODUCTION

The profession of communication sciences and disorders is in dire need of individuals to assist in the delivery of services to the increasing numbers of individuals from multicultural backgrounds with speech, language, or hearing problems. Individuals with bilingual skills are especially needed as audiologists and speech-language pathologists, and are mandated in many instances, to provide services in the native language(s) of their clients. Currently only about 2% of ASHA members are bilingual (see Figure 12-1).

All students interested in pursuing courses of study in these professions may want to consider the possibility of increasing their bilingual skills through participation in immersion programs and taking advanced courses in a foreign language. All students with multicultural or bilingual experiences and/or familiarity in working with racial/ethnic minority populations will be more marketable as these populations increase in numbers and become a larger proportion of the client population. This chapter discusses what students from culturally and linguistically diverse backgrounds can do to stay competitive, and Figure 12-2 offers a checklist to track your progress.

## Ask Questions About the Diversity of the Faculty and Students When Applying to an Academic Program

When investigating potential CSD programs, ask about diversity in both the faculty and the student population. Do not be afraid to ask these questions because it is important that you feel comfortable with the students you are going to network with and the professors who are going to train you for your career. Make sure that your graduate or undergraduate program is going to be a place that is supportive of students from culturally and linguistically diverse backgrounds.

**AMERICAN SPEECH-LANGUAGE-HEARING ASSOCIATION
SUMMARY MEMBERSHIP AND AFFILIATION COUNTS
JANUARY 1 THROUGH DECEMBER 31, 2003**

| Ethnicity | CCC in Speech | CCC in Audiology | Dual CCC | Certified Subtotal | In Process | Not Certified | Total |
|---|---|---|---|---|---|---|---|
| Hispanic or Latino | 1,587 | 133 | 7 | 1,727 | 18 | 18 | 1,763 |
| Not Hispanic or Latino | 55,954 | 6,894 | 595 | 63,443 | 402 | 347 | 64,192 |
| Not Specified | 40,412 | 5,789 | 781 | 46,982 | 853 | 245 | 48,080 |
| **Total** | 97,953 | 12,816 | 1,383 | 112,152 | 1,273 | 610 | 114,035 |

| Race | | | | | | | |
|---|---|---|---|---|---|---|---|
| American Indian/ Alaska Native (only) | 158 | 20 | 1 | 179 | 3 | 1 | 183 |
| Asian (only) | 825 | 179 | 14 | 1,018 | 17 | 31 | 1,066 |
| Black or African American (only) | 1,286 | 115 | 10 | 1,411 | 18 | 10 | 1,439 |
| Native Hawaiian/Other Pacific Islander (only) | 60 | 6 | 0 | 66 | 0 | 0 | 66 |
| White (only) | 54,020 | 6,566 | 558 | 61,144 | 374 | 303 | 61,821 |
| Multi-Racial | 1,191 | 149 | 20 | 1,360 | 10 | 19 | 1,389 |
| Not Specified | 40,413 | 5,781 | 780 | 46,974 | 851 | 246 | 48,071 |
| **Total** | 97,953 | 12,816 | 1,383 | 112,152 | 1,273 | 610 | 114,035 |

**Figure 12-1** ASHA membership counts by race and ethnicity *(Source: 2003 ASHA Omnibus Survey)*

## Maintain a Competitive Grade Point Average

It is important to maintain a strong GPA throughout your undergraduate study in order to be considered for entry into a graduate program. The more competitive programs may have a 3.5 GPA minimum requirement. For all students, having good grades will be the key to getting accepted into a program and receiving scholarships.

## Prepare for the GRE and the Praxis Examination

Students planning on attending graduate school must take the Graduate Record Examination (GRE) and receive a competitive score. Your standardized test

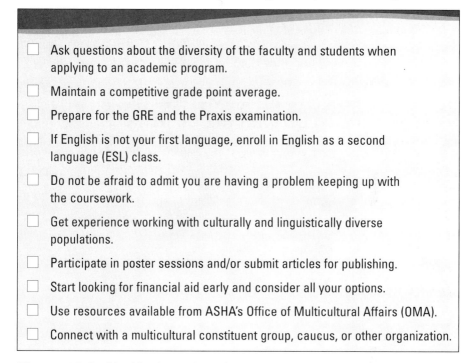

- [ ] Ask questions about the diversity of the faculty and students when applying to an academic program.

- [ ] Maintain a competitive grade point average.

- [ ] Prepare for the GRE and the Praxis examination.

- [ ] If English is not your first language, enroll in English as a second language (ESL) class.

- [ ] Do not be afraid to admit you are having a problem keeping up with the coursework.

- [ ] Get experience working with culturally and linguistically diverse populations.

- [ ] Participate in poster sessions and/or submit articles for publishing.

- [ ] Start looking for financial aid early and consider all your options.

- [ ] Use resources available from ASHA's Office of Multicultural Affairs (OMA).

- [ ] Connect with a multicultural constituent group, caucus, or other organization.

**Figure 12-2** Checklist for students from culturally and linguistically diverse backgrounds

scores will be a major factor in acceptance decisions for graduate schools, so prepare accordingly prior to taking those tests and make the most of any review courses or preparation programs that may be available. Similarly, prior to graduation from your graduate program you will be required to take either the Praxis examination in audiology or the Praxis examination in speech-language pathology for certification in the profession. Get whatever help you need to pass these exams. This is an investment in your future and you cannot afford to cut corners here. The National Black Association of Speech Language and Hearing (NBASLH) sponsors a Praxis review course for members twice each year. All students can join NBASLH to take advantage of the review courses.

## If English Is Not Your First Language, Enroll in English as a Second Language (ESL) Class

Most campuses and major cities have English as a second language (ESL) courses on campus or nearby for English language learners. These courses often include reading and writing skills enrichment. Let your professors know that English is not your first language and that you are continually working to improve your writing and speaking skills. Ask your faculty and peers for feedback on your progress in writing and speaking. Remember that proficiency in standard English, while generally not a specific requirement, will be an advantage in widening your range of clinical options after graduation. If you are an English language learner or speak a dialect other than standard English as your native dialect, take every opportunity to improve your standard English skills.

## Do Not Be Afraid to Admit You Are Having a Problem Keeping Up with the Coursework

If you are struggling with your coursework, especially if English is a second language, seek help. If needed, ask for additional time to complete assignments appropriately and accurately. Let your professor know that you are continually working to improve your English reading and writing skills. Ask your professor questions when you are unclear on an assignment's requirements. If allowed, work with a peer on assignments so that you can teach each other and complete assignments efficiently.

## Gain Experience Working with Culturally and Linguistically Diverse Populations

Once enrolled in your course of study, taking advantage of every opportunity to gain insight and expertise in the provision of services to multicultural populations will increase your potential contributions to the professions. During your breaks from school, consider volunteering in clinics in developing countries outside the United States. If this is not feasible, consider getting a summer job as a tutor for children who speak English as a second language, or working in a hospital where there is a diverse population.

## Participate in Poster Sessions and/or Submit Articles for Publishing

As you consider topics for assignments and projects, think about researching topics that are related to culturally and linguistically diverse populations. Use your research to add to the proliferation of research, assessment and therapeutic techniques, and philosophies relative to communication disorders within bilingual and minority populations. Share your work by participating in poster sessions at student conferences sponsored by your CSD department or in CSD departments of other schools, at state speech-language-hearing conventions, or during the NBASLH or ASHA convention. Also consider submitting papers to professional journals for publication.

## Start Looking for Financial Aid Early and Consider All Your Options

Your goal should be finding aid that will provide you with funding to meet all of your expenses. A number of academic programs are participating in campus-wide initiatives for increasing diversity and others simply have a desire to train professionals from racial/ethnic backgrounds. As a result, there may be scholarships, grants, or other forms of financial aid available specifically for ethnically and culturally diverse students. Ask your undergraduate or graduate program director about these funding opportunities.

## Use Resources Available from ASHA's Office of Multicultural Affairs (OMA)

ASHA has had a unit of the National Office devoted to diversity and multicultural issues for 35 years. ASHA's Office of Multicultural Affairs (OMA) provides technical assistance to its members and students in search of information and resources related to communication disorders in multicultural populations, as well as service delivery to those individuals. A detailed list of resources available from the OMA can be found on the ASHA Web site at http://www.asha. org.

## Connect with a Multicultural Constituent Group, Caucus, or Other Organization

There are a number of groups and organizations that provide support services to students. Figure 12-3 provides a list and brief description of each ASHA caucus and other organizations related to CLD populations.

## CONCLUSION

Audiologists and speech-language pathologists from culturally and linguistically diverse backgrounds are in strong demand to meet the needs of a growing multicultural population of individuals seeking services for speech, language, and hearing disorders. As a student from a culturally and/or linguistically diverse background, there are a number of resources available that are discussed in this chapter to help you achieve success in your undergraduate and graduate programs. By developing your CSD skills so they incorporate multicultural and multilinguistic abilities, you will find yourself well positioned for a successful career once you are ready for the job market.

## WORK CITED

American Speech-Language-Hearing Association. *2003 Omnibus survey: ASHA membership counts by race and ethnicity.* Rockville, MD, on the Internet at http://www.asha.org/members/research/reports/member-counts.htm (visited July 17, 2004).

Following is a list and brief description of each caucus or other organization related to CLD populations. Links to the ASHA-recognized Multicultural Constituency Groups is available in the Members Only section of the ASHA Web site.

**Native American Caucus**

The Native American Caucus addresses issues related to clients and professionals who are Native American. The caucus promotes awareness of Native American Culture.

**Hispanic Caucus**

The Hispanic Caucus discusses and addresses problems related to professionals, students, and clients who are Hispanic.

**Asian-Indian Caucus**

The Asian-Indian Caucus (AIC) promotes collaboration of knowledge and research about individuals who are Asian-Indian.

**Asian Pacific Islander Caucus**

The Asia Pacific Caucus works to increase the number of students who are Asian Pacific Islander (API) and discusses issues related to professionals, clients, and students who are API. This caucus works to increase other professions' awareness of working with API clients who are receiving audiology, speech, and/or language services.

**Lesbian/Gay/Bisexual Audiologists and Speech-Language Pathologists**

The Lesbian/Gay/Bisexual Audiologists and Speech-Language Pathologists (L'GASP) group provides a forum to discuss issues related to L'GASP's professional needs and concerns, such as addressing homophobia in the workplace.

**National Council of La Raza**

The National Council of La Raza (NCLR) works to increase opportunities and decrease discrimination and poverty among Hispanic Americans. NCLR has a Hispanic Scholarship Fund Institute for students who are Hispanic. Their Web site is http://www.nclr.org.

**National Black Association for Speech-Language and Hearing**

The National Black Association for Speech-Language and Hearing (NBASLH) addresses the issues related to professionals, students, and clients who are African American. Their Web site is http://www.nbaslh.org.

**ASHA Special Interest Division 14**

The ASHA Special Interest Division on Communication Disorders and Sciences in CLD Populations provides continuing education materials, networking opportunities, and mentoring opportunities for students.

**The National Black Graduate Student Association, Inc.**

The National Black Graduate Student Association, Inc. (NBGSA) works to address African American students' needs and concerns in college and graduate school. Their Web site is http://www.nbgsa.org.

**The Hispanic Scholarship Fund (HSF)**

The Hispanic Scholarship Fund is the nation's leading organization supporting Hispanic higher education and is committed to providing opportunities for students. For more information on the HSF, visit their Web site at http://www.hsf.net.

**Figure 12-3** Caucuses and other resources for culturally and linguistically diverse students

# CHAPTER 13

## Advice for Students with an Undergraduate Degree in Another Discipline

### INTRODUCTION

It is not uncommon for students to enter a graduate CSD program with an undergraduate degree in another discipline. Individuals who may have worked for several years in a different field often seek the CSD profession when making a career change. Many programs are very welcoming of students from different disciplines and backgrounds. In fact, if you have a degree in a related area (e.g., Linguistics, Education, Spanish), this makes you very enticing to graduate programs. Your unique perspective can aid in classroom discussions as well as in clinical work. Keep in mind that you will probably have to take one year of undergraduate CSD courses before taking graduate-level courses. This chapter discusses some other things you should consider, and Figure 13-1 provides a checklist to track your progress.

### Contact the CSD Department of Your Prospective Graduate Program

Ask to speak with the director of graduate studies and the undergraduate advisor in CSD to find out what undergraduate requirements you will need to fulfill. Consider asking the following questions:

- What courses will I need to take to graduate?
- How many credit hours will I need to graduate?
- How long does it usually take to complete the prerequisite coursework?
- What courses are required for teacher certification? (If you are considering working in a school, your state may require that you complete a certain number of education courses.)
- Will I need to take the prerequisite courses before I apply to the graduate program?
- Do I need to apply for the prerequisite courses?
- Who do I contact to discuss what courses from my undergraduate transcript will transfer?
- When are the courses typically scheduled (night, day, weekend)?
- Are any of the courses offered online?

- [ ] Contact the CSD department of your prospective graduate program.
- [ ] Ascertain the technical term your university uses for students in your position.
- [ ] Take some undergraduate prerequisites during the summer.
- [ ] Observe a professional in the field.
- [ ] Expect to take one year to complete most of the undergraduate coursework.
- [ ] Get to know other "post-bachs."
- [ ] Learn good time management skills.
- [ ] Make time for fun and relaxation.
- [ ] Make time for sleep.
- [ ] Limit outside work, if possible.
- [ ] Talk with students taking junior- and senior-level classes.
- [ ] Join NSSLHA.
- [ ] Become involved with your local chapter of NSSLHA.
- [ ] Identify the unique qualities that you bring to class.
- [ ] When things get tough, remember your goals.

**Figure 13-1** Checklist for students with an undergraduate degree in another discipline

## Ascertain the Technical Term Your University Uses for Students in Your Position

Some universities use "post-bachs," "prerequisites," or "deficiencies" when referring to students in a CSD graduate program with a different major. Although the terms are synonymous, you should use your program's jargon.

## Take Some Undergraduate Prerequisites During the Summer

If possible, try to get a jump start on undergraduate prerequisites during the summer before your first year in a graduate program. This will help transition you into full-time CSD coursework and it may lighten your class load.

## Observe a Professional in the Field

If you have not done so already, observing a professional audiologist or speech-language pathologist will help you evaluate if you can truly picture yourself as a clinician. Ask the clinical director at the program you plan to attend to refer you to a former post-bachelor student who you could observe and speak with about his or her academic experience. These hours are to help you learn more about the profession and are separate from ASHA's required observation hours; most programs require observations as requirements of specific classes.

## Expect to Take One Year to Complete Most of the Undergraduate Coursework

Undergraduates who major in CSD usually take two years of courses within their major. It will most likely take you one year to take all the CSD prerequisites needed before you begin graduate study.

## Get to Know Other "Post-Bachs"

Only prerequisite students know what it is truly like to take 20 credit hours of CSD courses in a semester. Prerequisite students have a special bond that only prerequisites can understand. Share your experiences with other prerequisites. Exchange stories about the career path you took, or almost took. Developing relationships with students with similar interests can lead to a great support system of people to study, observe, and work on projects with; you may find these relationships follow you through your graduate work.

## Learn Good Time Management Skills

You will need to balance your time wisely to complete assignments on time and prepare for exams. If you have been a procrastinator in the past, this is a great time to overcome it. If you need help developing time management skills, find out if your school offers courses through a learning center or academic advising office. You can also search the library or a bookstore for resources.

## Make Time for Fun and Relaxation

Even though you are busy with class work and possibly clinical work, you have to make room for downtime. At least once a week, do something fun or relaxing. Watch a movie with friends, go dancing, go to your place of worship, play Frisbee, take a yoga class, or read a novel. Continue to be an active member of the community. Relax whenever you have the opportunity, especially over long weekends and spring break.

## Make Time for Sleep

Find a way to balance your study time and sleep schedule. Most people learn and function most efficiently when they are well rested. Make sleep a priority.

## Limit Outside Work, If Possible

Trying to balance a full-time course load, studying, a full-time job, personal/social time, and sleep is quite difficult—and for many it seems impossible. Understandably, you may need to work for financial reasons. If working while being a full-time student is too overwhelming, look into student loans and other financial assistance. If possible, try to work only part-time to make your schedule more manageable. If this is not possible, consider taking courses part-time if that is an option in your program.

## Talk with Students Taking
## Junior- and Senior-Level Classes

Ask undergraduate juniors and seniors in your classes what they think of the courses. For instance, ask the seniors for advice on some of the junior-level classes. They may have insight about classes or sections that were particularly useful, or may have recommendations about professors who are particularly strong instructors.

## Join NSSLHA

The membership benefits and access to journals and online resources will quickly familiarize you with current events in the profession. Refer back to Chapter 3 to learn more about the many benefits of joining NSSLHA.

## Become Involved with Your
## Local Chapter of NSSLHA

Joining your local NSSLHA chapter is a great way to become an active member of your school's CSD community and to learn more about the profession. You can get to know your classmates at social events and become involved with volunteer activities. Refer back to Chapter 3 for more information on local NSSLHA chapters.

## Identify the Unique Qualities That You Bring to Class

It may be frustrating to have an undergraduate degree and still be taking undergraduate classes. Use your experience to help other students in your courses and enrich your own educational experience. What skills have you gained from your first undergraduate degree that you can use in CSD? For example, someone with a degree in special education is familiar with the Individuals with Disabilities Education Act (IDEA) and Individual Education Plans (IEPs) that are required by law. Share your relevant experiences with the class.

## When Things Get Tough, Remember Your Goals

Hard work in graduate school will lead to greater payoffs in the future. Picture yourself as a successful therapist/scientist whenever you doubt your abilities or are feeling overwhelmed by the demands on your time. A positive attitude is the key to a promising future. If you are passionate about the field and believe in yourself, you will make it through.

## CONCLUSION

Students with majors in fields other than CSD can most certainly obtain a graduate degree in audiology or speech-language pathology, but the road to a successful career will be a little longer than for traditional CSD majors. However, you bring to your studies all the knowledge you gained from your first major, which can give you a valuable perspective on issues in CSD and may translate to an even more successful professional practice. Use this chapter to help identify actions you will need to take to get the most out of your prerequisite courses and to transition smoothly into graduate coursework.

# CHAPTER 14

# Transitioning from Undergraduate to Graduate Coursework

Marie A. Patton, master's student, SLP, University of Wisconsin-Madison and NSSLHA President, 2001-2003

## INTRODUCTION

Whether your graduate program is two, three, or five years, you will have much information to learn in a relatively short amount of time. Fortunately, faculty members do not expect you to learn everything there is to know about the field of communication sciences and disorders during this time. Instead, your graduate study will be the time to learn the tools and techniques to work with clients and conduct research. Once you graduate, you will fine tune your clinical and research skills while working.

Students who transition from undergraduate to graduate programs soon discover that being a graduate student is much more challenging than being an undergraduate. Graduate students have to learn to think differently, adjust to new ways of assessment, write more frequently, and manage their time better. This chapter offers advice from Geralyn M. Schulz, PhD, CCC-SLP, the Chair of the Communication Sciences program at George Washington University, on students transitioning from an undergraduate to a graduate CSD program. Marie Patton also offers advice on the transition, as this chapter was written during her first year of graduate study.

## There Can Be Many Right Answers to Problems

Most undergraduate courses use true/false and multiple choice tests where there is only one correct answer to each question. Students are used to memorizing material, recognizing the "right" answers, and regurgitating what was taught. When these students enter graduate school, they soon discover that there is more than one "right" answer to a problem. In CSD, the "right" answer may vary based on the case; the severity of a disorder; the client's personal, social, psychological, financial, religious, and cultural concerns; or increasingly, on what insurance or Medicare/Medicaid will cover. Likewise, within the field there are differing philosophies or theories of assessment, diagnosis and treatment, and depending on the theoretical approach, the "right" answer to a problem may vary widely.

## You Know More Than You Think You Know

Faculty members prefer students to express their ideas, as long as the student has a reason for what he or she is saying. Sometimes when a faculty member asks a student a challenging question, the student may respond, "I don't know because I have not taken a class on it yet." This type of response may cause frustration to both the student and faculty member. Instead of focusing on what he or she *does not* yet know, a student should always try to answer the question based upon what he or she *does* know. Furthermore, a student can follow up an answer by stating how to find out more information or ask the faculty member a specific question that will help lead to a solution.

Much like the experiences students face in graduate school when approaching a new topic for the first time, clinicians and researchers will be faced with situations that are unfamiliar to them. However, those who pull from their previous knowledge and ask questions are more likely to effectively solve problems. Like students, faculty members reason and think their way through right and wrong possibilities. The sooner students realize that they need to consider several right answers, the more likely they will provide good care for their clients and solve research questions.

## You Are Assessed Differently

Professors in graduate courses usually assess students' knowledge by giving essay or short answer exams, case studies, group assignments, and papers. Some papers may be twenty or thirty pages in length, which is considerably longer than the types of papers written in undergraduate courses. Other papers may be limited to one page, but must be written very concisely. Graduate classes are more likely to be interactive. Students are expected to ask questions and discuss assigned readings and material presented in class. Some courses may have a lab component. In many clinical practica, students are assessed according to their interactions with their clients, preparation for sessions, and written reports. Unlike undergraduate courses, professors are less likely to use multiple choice and short answer tests.

## You Are Not, and Cannot Be, Perfect

Students who go through their undergraduate programs with 4.0 grade point averages and are at the top of their class may become accustomed to "being right all of the time." When these students enter graduate school and are told that they did something wrong in clinic, they may not know how to react. As a result, they may become overly stressed because they are used to performing "perfectly" and are struggling to achieve that same level of perfection. For their own sanity and for the sake of others, students should realize that they are not, and cannot be, perfect at everything.

Students who are trying to act "perfect" all the time are likely to exude their attitude, often indirectly, on their clients. Clients can pick up on their clinicians' perfectionism and feel burdened that they have to be perfect as well.

## You Are Not Expected to Know as Much as Your Professors

Students should not expect themselves to know as much as their professors. Professors should know more than the students because the professors may have taken 10 to 30 years to get where they are. Students should be patient with themselves and appreciate that they can learn from their professors, just as one day soon, they will learn from their co-workers and clients.

## Collaborate with Your Classmates

During undergraduate studies, many students are competitive with their classmates because they are striving to get a spot in their prospective graduate program. Many students feel that they need to be better than others in order to get into graduate school. However, once in graduate school, students should let go of this competitiveness. Most clinicians will not be competing for the same jobs. Plus, graduate school is much easier when students work together as a team and support each other as friends and colleagues.

## Constantly Improve Your Time Management Skills

As the saying goes, "if you want to get something done, give it to a busy person." Students who are good at planning are usually less critical of themselves and complete assignments without undue stress. Students who do not manage their time may find themselves completing assignments at the last minute and will wish they had more time to do a better job.

Undergraduate students who balanced school, work, a job, volunteer work, a family, and/or extracurricular activities (e.g., NSSLHA, band, sport team), are going to adjust better to graduate school than other students. Graduate students should not expect to have the same lifestyle that many undergraduates have of going out most nights.

To avoid procrastination, students should improve their planning skills. In graduate school, it is quite unlikely that a student will have a whole day to complete a single assignment. Instead of waiting until six hours before a lengthy assignment is due, students should work on assignments in smaller increments. They should take advantage of the fifteen minutes between classes or twenty minutes on the bus to get work done. In fifteen or twenty minutes, students can probably write a goal for a therapy report or learn a page of notes. This useful skill can generalize to other situations. For example, those who are married and have a family are unlikely to have a large chunk of time to complete any lengthy task. Professors also struggle with not having a large amount of time to prepare for courses, work on research, and meet with students. Students should adjust to completing tasks in small increments now, rather than later.

The struggles that students experience from transitioning from undergraduate to graduate coursework are normal. Many students have difficulty because their free time is taken away. Students should realize that graduate school can be a 60 to 80 hour-per-week job. The main difference is that most students pay for the experience instead of getting paid. To be successful, graduate school requires a lot of work outside of class.

As most first-year graduate students will notice, the number of credit hours for a full-time load is less than it is for undergraduate studies. However, in graduate school, students will spend more time per credit hour than they did in undergraduate courses. Some variation in the amount of time spent occurs in graduate school among the types of classes. For many students, the most time-consuming part of their course load is their clinical experience. Sometimes, being enrolled for only one credit hour of clinic can take up as much time as a three-credit-hour graduate class. This is because a beginning clinician will take a lot of time to plan for sessions, gather and/or create materials, prepare for meetings with a clinical instructor, and write reports. With experience, student clinicians will decrease the amount of time they spend preparing for clinic and writing reports.

## Relax: Most Students Make It Through

Students should be comforted in knowing that it is extremely rare that someone does not make it through graduate school. These very few who do not make it through usually decide to take a different career path because the clinical experience was not what they thought it would be. These students usually did not have an undergraduate clinical practicum experience, and sometimes choose to go into research psychology or another field without clinical practicum, but still related to healthcare. It is extremely rare for students to not make it through graduate school because of academic grades.

Students also need to realize that in graduate school, decisions are rarely "life and death." Audiology and speech-language pathology are not like surgery. In general, clinical experiences are only extremely critical situations when working in intensive care or with patients who have dysphagia. Fortunately, when clinically-related decisions need to be made that may result in life or death outcomes, student will be working with experienced supervisors. The supervisors will teach them how to sort through the difficult decisions they face.

## CONCLUSION

Transitioning from undergraduate to graduate coursework is challenging. Learning to problem solve, being more confident, getting used to the ways of assessment, striving to do well (while appreciating that perfection is unrealistic), and working with classmates can help students make a smooth transition. Students should keep in mind that every year, graduate students successfully transition from undergraduate to graduate coursework in audiology and speech-language pathology. Students should try to enjoy their time in graduate school. It will go by more quickly than expected.

# CHAPTER 15

# Research Basics

Marie A. Patton, master's student, SLP, University of
Wisconsin-Madison and NSSLHA President, 2001-2003

## INTRODUCTION

As an undergraduate or as a graduate student, you have probably heard about the projected doctoral shortages nationwide. The "graying of CSD faculty" will soon lead to many Ph.D.-level positions being left unfilled as more faculty members retire. The field needs new researchers to replace those who will retire. Does research interest you? Hopefully, this chapter will help you consider going into research, how to get involved in research, and how to be a successful researcher. Based upon a discussion with Ray Kent, a Professor at the University of Wisconsin-Madison and ASHA Vice President for Research and Technology (2004-2007), the following are some tips to determine if research is the career for you.

## Ask a Professor If You Can Be Involved with a Research Project

Ask your professors what they are researching. If a project interests you, ask if the professor has any paying positions as an assistant available. This could be a great way to help fund your education and learn about research at the same time. If there are no paying positions, ask if the professor could use volunteer assistance. The experience gained working with a seasoned professor on a topic that really interests you could be priceless.

## Take a Course in Research

If your department offers a course in research, take it! If not, check for a discipline-wide research course.

## Attend Sessions About Research at Conferences and Conventions

The ASHA Convention offers various sessions related to research. Usually in the springtime, ASHA hosts a research conference on communication disorders.

Some state conventions offer research sessions. By attending these sessions you will see how different researchers formulate research questions, set up studies, and present their findings.

## Choose a Topic to Research Based Upon What Interests You

When you take CSD courses, make note of questions the professors or authors of your textbooks say have not been researched or have not been answered. Outside of class, read about areas that spark your interest. Moreover, you can find research questions at the end of journal articles where the authors discuss further research questions that need to be answered. When you find a topic that interests you, try to work it into projects for your different graduate courses.

## Take a Grant Writing Course

If a grant writing course is available at your university, take it. Doctoral programs will usually address grant writing within the department. The course typically explains how to choose human participants within the guidelines of the Institutional Review Board; ethics; funding agencies; and how to write the review of literature, procedures, and methods in detail within the page limits.

Researchers do not always use only one funding source. For instance, a researcher may get seed money from a smaller funding source, such as the March of Dimes, and then seek support from the National Institute on Deafness and other Communication Disorders (NICHD).

A grant writing course will probably explain the process of approving a grant. Here is a brief overview of the grant review process at the National Institute of Health (NIH), NIDCD, and NICHD:

- Submit your grant to one of the NIH study sessions that are offered three times per year.
- At least two reviewers read, discuss, and score your grant. The reviewers evaluate grants on a scale of one to five, based upon which grants have the highest significance. The lower the number, the better the score. If a grant has too many flaws, an "NS," or no score, is given.
- If the grant receives a one or a two, an advisory council who approves funding reviews the grant. The council identifies grants that address areas related to human health that have been neglected. The advisory council who reviews CSD-related grants can consist of otolaryngologists, neuroscientists, biological scientists, psychologists, linguists, professionals in CSD, and some public members related to the professions.

# After Completing Your Research, Choose a Journal for Submission

Your results and discussion sections can lead you to which outlet would be best suited to publish your research findings. Choose a journal based upon the audience who reads the journal. The goal is to have your research findings impact the largest number of clinicians and researchers who would benefit from knowing your research findings.

## Get a Post Doctorate

A post doctorate is a full-time research position that usually lasts between one and three years. The post doctorate is a valuable research apprenticeship and basically is the only time that a researcher can conduct research without having other duties. For instance, a professor has to balance research, teaching, and committee duties. Except for a sabbatical, a post doctorate is the only time a researcher can be fully devoted to research. Also, a post doctorate will gain more research and grantsmanship experience with a mentor, which will enhance research skills and marketability when applying for faculty positions or other jobs. Usually, those with a post doctorate are paid higher than those with only a doctorate. Interestingly, other science fields, like physics and biology, expect researchers to have a post doctorate before beginning a research position. Read Chapter 24 for more information on post doctorates.

## Read Journal Articles Outside of Class

The *Journal of Speech, Language, and Hearing Research* (JSLHR) combines clinic and research on a variety of topics in CSD and would be a good journal to read on a regular basis. The journal includes position papers, scientific investigations, and clinical studies. JSLHR is considered by some to be the best journal in the field. Additional journal selections are available in the special interest sections of the *Survival Guide*. The following is a list of journals that ASHA publishes:

- *American Journal of Audiology* (AJA)
- *American Journal of Speech-Language Pathology* (AJSLP)
- *Journal of Speech, Language, and Hearing Research* (JSLHR)
- *Language, Speech, and Hearing Services in Schools* (LSHSS)

## Develop Qualities of a Good Researcher

Learn the qualities needed to be a good researcher, and develop them if you do not already possess them:

- Creativity
- Commitment

- Tenacity
- Diligence
- Value interacting with others (e.g., at conferences)
- Enjoy publishing
- Love for knowledge

## CONCLUSION

Research is the basis from which new assessments, diagnoses, and treatments are derived and is fundamentally important to the growth of knowledge about communication sciences and disorders. If research interests you, create your own opportunities at the graduate and post-graduate levels to hone your skills, perform valuable work, and share your findings with the community at large.

# CHAPTER 16

# Writing a Thesis

## INTRODUCTION

Writing a thesis is a great introduction to research and may assist you in deciding if research is something you want to pursue as a career. Many master's students write a thesis because they plan to continue their education at the doctoral level. In many doctoral programs, students who did not write a master's thesis must complete one when they begin the doctoral program. Writing a thesis as a doctoral student prolongs the doctoral program. However, in other programs, students write a "predissertation" regardless of writing a thesis, where students independently pilot research and publish the research in a peer-reviewed journal.

In some master's programs, the tract for writing a thesis is clear cut. For instance, the program may have a research methods course, where the thesis is explained and chapters of the thesis are written. For other master's programs, students learn about the thesis from their advisor or research mentor and then write it independently or take thesis credit hours. This chapter applies mainly to students whose graduate programs reflect the latter scenario.

Realize that writing a thesis may be the most challenging academic experience you will have to date. However, writing a thesis may be the most rewarding experience you will have as a master's student. This chapter offers advice as you work on your thesis, and Figure 16-1 is a checklist you can use to track your progress.

## Identify a Topic Area

Choose a topic based upon the area in the field of communication sciences and disorders that interests you the most. At this point, you do not have to know the exact research question(s) you will address in your thesis; think general rather than specific. Your research mentor and committee (explained later in this chapter) will assist you with the exact research question or questions for your thesis. However, be certain about the area you want to study. You will be devoting at least a year of intense research to the topic. If you are not highly interested in a topic and choose one because an advisor tells you to do so, you will find it difficult to complete the thesis. Ask yourself:

- Why am I interested in this topic?
- Did this phenomenon affect a client or family member?

- ☐ Identify a topic area.
- ☐ Identify a mentor for your thesis.
- ☐ Consider whether to interview your own participants or use previously collected data.
- ☐ Complete and submit the human participant's permission form.
- ☐ Realize that it is unrealistic to complete a longitudinal study during your 2- to 3-year master's program.
- ☐ Form a thesis committee.
- ☐ Register for thesis credit each semester you work on your thesis.
- ☐ Know and observe all thesis deadlines.
- ☐ Consider taking a statistics course.
- ☐ Review the literature on your topic.
- ☐ Write the proposal for your thesis.
- ☐ Find out what style you should use.
- ☐ Submit your proposal to the thesis committee when it is complete.
- ☐ Complete your thesis when your proposal is approved.
- ☐ Defend your completed thesis.
- ☐ Follow your university's requirements for having the thesis catalogued and bound.
- ☐ Submit your research as a poster presentation or formal presentation.
- ☐ Submit your thesis for publication.

**Figure 16-1** Checklist for writing a thesis

- Did I first become interested in this topic because of a class that I had?
- What aspects of this topic interest me the most?
- What do I need to learn about this topic before I choose to use it for my thesis?
- What experiences can I have now that would prepare me to research any topic?
- What research experiences or projects have I completed in my undergraduate coursework that may help me if I write my thesis on this topic?

# Identify a Mentor for Your Thesis

Choose a mentor based upon a research area that interests you. Refer to the department Web page, ask classmates, and/or ask your advisor which professor in the department researches your topic area. Depending on your topic, you may find that no one in your department shares your interest. You may have to change your topic, or find a mentor whose research interests most closely match your own.

Once you find a professor who researches in your topic, make contact by phone or email. Inform the professor that you are interested in writing a thesis, and would like to pursue a doctorate (if that is true). Request a meeting to learn more about the professor's research and discuss the possibility of writing your thesis on the topic.

*Prior to the appointment with a potential research mentor:*

- Prepare questions to ask the professor by looking up journal articles, textbooks, or textbook chapters that the professor has recently published on the topic. Reading the professor's work will give you a better understanding of what he or she does and allow you to ask the professor questions about the research (which makes you look well prepared).

- Have a general idea of the direction you would like to take your research. This may not be the direction you finally take, but the professor may have questions for you about your potential thesis. It will help the professor make an informed decision about working with you if you are able to articulate your area of interest.

*During the appointment:*

- Ask the potential research mentor what he or she is currently researching.

- Consider asking if the professor has been a mentor to other students who have written a thesis.

- Inquire about thesis guidelines or a handbook that describes the entire process involved in writing a thesis in your department. It is very important that you become aware of your university and department requirements and timelines. Often, this information will also be available on your university's Web site.

- Ask what areas within your chosen topic you should research.

*During and after the appointment:*

- Evaluate how well you think you would interact with the professor if you had to work together for at least the next year. Is he or she easy to talk to, knowledgeable about the topic, and available to be a research mentor? Has he or she ever chaired a thesis committee before?

- Ask if the professor would like to be your primary research mentor for your thesis, if it seems like a good match for you. Most students have difficulty identifying a specific question to research because they have not yet learned enough about the general topic to know what questions have not been investigated. Your mentor should be knowledgeable enough about the topic to help. In fact, you may be asked to take on a small part of a project that the professor is working on, but does not have time to explore.

- If your areas of interest do not seem well suited, or if the professor does not have time to be an effective mentor, ask for suggestions of other professors in the department who may be a better fit for you and your project.

## Consider Whether to Interview Your Own Participants or Use Previously Collected Data

If you use data that has already been collected by another researcher (e.g., faculty member at your university or another university) as the basis for your thesis, you could save yourself months of valuable time. Although the choice is up to you, remember that you will most likely interview your own participants when you write your dissertation in a doctoral program.

If you choose to select your own participants, the first thing you have to do is find them. Ask your clinic director if he or she knows of eligible participants. You can also contact any support groups in your area, or you could contact clinical faculty or local clinicians. Realize that even finding two participants may be challenging and time consuming depending on your selection criteria. Thus, after your proposal has been approved, start searching for participants right away.

## Complete and Submit the Human Participants Permission Form

If you plan to use your own participants, you must complete and submit the human participants permission form to the Institutional Review Board (IRB) to seek their approval, prior to contacting your participants. Ask your research mentor how and when to begin the process. It is your responsibility to complete the forms and turn them in on time. Find out the dates for when the IRB meets and when to submit papers. Some IRBs only meet once each month. Try to seek IRB approval several months before you plan on selecting participants. You may need to revise your thesis before the IRB will approve it. Seek advice from your research mentor because he or she has probably had a lot of experience in having projects approved by the IRB.

# Realize That It Is Unrealistic to Complete a Longitudinal Study During Your 2- to 3-Year Master's Program

Longitudinal studies collect data on participants over a period of years. Do not bite off more than you can chew with your first major research project. Planning a longitudinal study for your master's research project will not allow you time to discuss results in your thesis, and may lead to complications with passing or approving the thesis. It is possible this could hold up the completion of your master's program and delay your graduation.

# Form a Thesis Committee

Most academic programs require a thesis committee. Your mentor will be the chair of the committee and should help you form this committee, which typically has two or three faculty members in your department. Sometimes, a professor from an outside department is asked to join the committee. Members should either be knowledgeable about the topic that you will research or have special expertise to contribute, such as statistical analysis. Some academic programs do not start the thesis process until the second year of study. If this is the case at your university, start developing good relationships with potential committee members early.

# Register for Thesis Credit Each Semester You Work on Your Thesis

Some programs may require academic credit for work on a thesis. Ask your department chair or research mentor about registration requirements at your university.

# Know and Observe All Thesis Deadlines

It is your responsibility to know and observe all deadlines and required paperwork associated with your thesis. It is up to you to schedule meetings, ensure that required forms are filed on time, and disseminate manuscripts to all committee members. Set realistic timelines. Realize that not everything will run smoothly, especially if you are conducting subject selection and participation. Have a contingency plan and be flexible.

# Consider Taking a Statistics Course

If you have not taken a statistics course yet, or if you would like to enhance your statistical skills, register for one. Having a good grasp on statistics will enhance your thesis experience right from the start. You will be required to take statistic courses as a doctoral student. Ask your research mentor if you should take a statistics course, and what course is recommended.

## Review the Literature on Your Topic

If you are not efficient at finding journal articles through your university's library or Web site, go to the library on campus that is related to CSD, such as the Health Sciences or Medical library, and ask a librarian to show you how to look up journal articles. Some universities offer one-time, non-credit, mini-courses on researching journal articles—take advantage of these courses. Moreover, ask your mentor for recommendations on journal articles and text book chapters you should read. If you find a great article or chapter on your topic, use the accompanying reference list or bibliography as a starting point for your research. These references may not be the most recent, but they can provide a solid foundation of understanding for your topic.

## Write the Proposal for Your Thesis

Ask your research mentor when you should start the thesis proposal process. The proposal typically consists of the first three chapters of the thesis, and includes the literature review, statement of the problem and research questions/hypotheses, and research methodology. However, many departments have slightly different formats for the proposal, so ask about your department's requirements.

Ask your advisor for previous thesis projects he or she has overseen. These will give you ideas for the general layout, grammar, literature review, and other formats that can help you get started. You may want to refer to the book, *Dissertations and Theses from Start to Finish: Psychology and Related Fields* by John D. Cone and Sharon L. Foster (1993).

Know that your committee will read your proposal. It is your responsibility to prepare a proposal that is free from errors, including grammar, spelling, organization, and presentation or layout. Committee members should be able to devote themselves to the project's content and not be expected to do significant editing. Have a friend edit the proposal or consider contacting someone from the campus writing center for feedback.

## Find Out What Style You Should Use

In most CSD departments in the U.S., the most recent edition of the *Publication Manual of the American Psychological Association* (APA) is used for style guidelines. The *APA Publications Manual* is a useful resource for learning the APA style. Find out what the preferred style for your program is and stick to it.

# Submit Your Proposal to the Thesis Committee When It Is Complete

When you have completed your thesis proposal, submit it to your thesis committee. The committee will review your proposal and provide helpful feedback to make sure that you have a successful thesis experience. In many programs, there is a formal meeting during which you will orally "defend" your proposal. This means that you present a summary of your work and answer questions. You may be asked to leave the room while committee members vote on the proposal. The proposal may be approved at this time. Be ready for possible rewrites. Depending on your writing style and knowledge of what a thesis entails, you may be resubmitting your proposal several times.

# Complete Your Thesis When Your Proposal is Approved

Once your proposal is approved, do not wait to get started finishing the thesis. Collect data, analyze results, and write the discussion chapters.

# Defend Your Completed Thesis

When you have completed your thesis, you will most likely need to defend it to your thesis committee and possibly others, such as the department chair, faculty members, and students. Talk with your research mentor or advisor about this process so you will know what to expect. Know and follow any departmental or university-wide procedures for completing this step.

# Follow Your University's Requirements for Having the Thesis Catalogued and Bound

Most universities permanently store a copy of every thesis in the library. Your university may have special requirements for how your thesis is presented, copied, and bound. Know and follow these requirements.

# Submit Your Research as a Poster Presentation or Formal Presentation

Now that you have completed your research and successfully defended it, share your work with others by presenting a poster presentation or formal presentation at a state or national convention. Many state associations encourage students to give poster presentations. Contact your state association to find out the deadline for submission and what is required. Deadlines for spring conventions may be due the summer prior to the convention. Applications for poster presentations for the ASHA Convention are usually due in April. Check the ASHA Web site for more detailed instructions on how to apply for the "Call for Papers," or CFP.

## Submit Your Thesis for Publication

Research finds practical applications only once it is shared with the professional community. Share your work with your colleagues by submitting it for publication in a scholarly journal. Since your research mentor typically puts a great deal of effort into helping you produce a quality thesis, you should be aware that it is customary, but not obligatory, to include him or her as a second author of any resulting publication or presentation.

NSSLHA's scholarly journal *Contemporary Issues in Communication Sciences and Disorders* (CICSD) accepts student papers for publication. Visit the information for authors section on the publication page of the NSSLHA Web site to learn more about the procedures for submitting articles for publication. You will also find information on the CICSD Mentoring Program that will pair students and first time authors with a research mentor who can assist with writing a paper for publication. NSSLHA awards an honorarium for student papers accepted for publication.

## CONCLUSION

If you chose to write a thesis, you will embark on what will likely be one of the more challenging and rewarding experiences of your academic career. It may be the only major research project you engage in if you go directly into clinical practice following graduation with your master's degree, or it may be just the start of a long career of professional research and publication. It is very important to remember that the practices outlined in this chapter covers only the general process for researching, writing, and defending a thesis. Check with your program for information on the process as it applies to you specifically, and then follow that procedure exactly. With all the incredible time, effort, thought, and writing you will be putting into this significant undertaking, you do not want to find your thesis (and possibly your graduation) is held up due to misfiled paperwork, improperly followed procedures, or some other clerical error.

# CHAPTER 17

# Writing for the Clinical Practicum

Michelle Cox, MA, Cinthia Gannett, Ph.D., Amy Solomon
Plante, M.S., CCC-SLP, and Jeanne O'Sullivan, M.Ed., CCC-SLP*

## INTRODUCTION

When we think of the professional work of speech-language pathologists, we often think of therapy—the face-to-face contact with clients. While the therapy is important, clinical writing is equally important to a client's program. Once the semester is over, only clinical documentation and reports remain to tell the story of what took place during therapy—the amount of progress a client achieved, how quickly a client progressed toward a goal, what did and did not work, what kinds of activities held the client's attention, and what the client liked to talk about.

As one of the main modes of communication between you and others who are involved in the client's treatment, such as parents, teachers, health care providers and caretakers, clinical writing has a valuable role in supporting a client's treatment. The reports we write educate others about what we are doing, what we have done, and ways others might support and supplement treatment. These reports also serve to prepare the next clinician, as the pieces you add to your client's chart provide information that is critical to developing a treatment plan that supports and builds upon the work already done.

Clinical writing is also important for you, as a student and developing professional. Composing reports not only documents services, but also affords you the opportunity to construct knowledge and apply what you are learning about the field and about your client. The treatment plan is the place for you to think through the goals and the steps you will take to get there. The progress report gives you a space to pull together and reflect on a semester's worth of treatment and experiences. Many of the readers of your clinical writing will not meet you in person, so your writing serves as a way for you to begin to establish your professional identity. For these readers, you *are* your writing.

*Ms. Cox is a Doctorate of Philosophy candidate in Composition Studies at the University of New Hampshire. Dr. Gannett is Director of Writing across the Curriculum at Loyola College. Dr. Plante is a Clinical Assistant Professor at the University of New Hampshire. Dr. Sullivan is a Clinical Assistant Professor at the University of New Hampshire.*

The University of New Hampshire (UNH) has been studying clinical writing and clinical writing instruction since 1998. This research started when clinical faculty initiated collaboration with the Writing Across the Curriculum (WAC) program, which is devoted to supporting faculty in developing writing curriculum. This chapter emerges from observations of those aspects of clinical writing that students most often struggle with, as well as techniques used to support student writing. We begin by identifying rhetorical aspects of clinical writing, such as genre, stakes, audiences, and readability, and suggest strategies for using rhetorical awareness to facilitate the writing process.

Next, aspects of writing clinical reports that are particularly difficult to negotiate, such as reporting "good news" and "bad news," handling background information, writing objectives, and ways to negotiate these aspects of writing are discussed. Keep in mind that the strategies offered may not be applicable to writing in every practicum setting. For example, we often suggest revising documents after receiving feedback from supervisors or peers. However, in some settings, deadlines are so tight that a long revision process is not possible. Hopefully, the suggested strategies can be adapted to fit different situations. The chapter ends with a list and discussion of resources that graduate students can seek out to support their writing during their practicum experiences.

This chapter focuses on clinical writing in the area of speech-language pathology *rather than* audiology. There are some similarities in writing between each of these professions, however, depending on the clinical setting and genre. Some of the strategies described may be useful to audiology students as they explore writing conventions that are specific to their discipline.

## CLINICAL GENRES

When you write for the clinical practicum, you will write in a variety of clinical genres, including both clinical documentation and clinical reports (Figure 17-1). Clinical documentation refers to shorter, more routine writing, such as daily logs, lesson plans, attendance records, and SOAP notes (Subjective, Objective, Assessment, and Plan notes primarily used in a medical setting). Clinical reports are longer, more detailed documents that may be sent to a variety of audiences. These reports include treatment plans, progress reports, and diagnostic reports. Each of these genres can vary in length, format, and appearance depending on the clinical setting. The clinical documentation and report writing that you learn during the on-campus practicum will not always directly transfer to writing for off-campus practicum settings. For example, the long, detailed treatment plan written for the on-campus practicum may not be appropriate in a school setting, where the Individualized Educational Plan (IEP) serves the same purpose. As a student, it is essential to be aware that you will need to investigate writing practices at each of your practicum settings. You may want to bring copies of clinical writing from your on-campus practicum to initial meetings with off-campus clinical supervisors to use as a prompt to discuss writing conventions at that setting.

| Clinical Documentation | Description | Function |
|---|---|---|
| **Objectives** (Benchmarks, Goals, Functional Outcomes) | Specific goals around which treatment is based. The traditional form requires that the objectives be measurable and objective. Standard components are: <br> • *Skill:* the target behavior/competency. <br> • *Conditions:* the situations and degree of support anticipated for the individual to successfully demonstrate the skill. <br> • *Criteria:* a quantitative or qualitative means of tracking progress. The anticipated degree of success and independence the individual will achieve. | • Identify areas of priority to be addressed in treatment. <br> • Provide a vision for what is to be accomplished to improve the individual's communication skills. <br> • Afford a means for measuring growth. |
| **Daily Notes** (Lesson Plans, SOAP Notes, Progress Notes, Consultation Note, Assessment/ Treatment Checklists) | A record of each treatment session. May take a variety of forms depending on the setting. These are very brief notations that basically document that the service was provided, along with some information on progress with respect to treatment goals. | • Verifies that an individual received treatment. <br> • Date is always required. <br> • Time of day and length of session may also be mandated. <br> • Tracks progress. <br> • May include plans for the next session. |
| **Annual Treatment Plans** (Individualized Family Service Plan [IFSP] for early intervention, Individualized Educational Plan [IEP] for school age, Individualized Service Plan [ISP] for adults) | A collaborative document that outlines an array of services and supports. Written for and by families with input from any relevant disciplines. Includes starting points and end points for intervention on a yearly basis. | • Ensures that children and adults with disabilities will receive appropriate support services under guidelines established by federal law. <br> • A type of contract that outlines information on an individual's needs and how they will be addressed. |
| **Insurance Forms** | Forms submitted to third-party payers. Generally include clients' personal data, as well as numerical codes for type of problem and service, along with dates and times. | • Allows for reimbursement for services. |
| **Daily Records** (Attendance Logs, Clinical Hours, Schedules) | These records document the amount of time the clinician and client spend in therapy, and track appointments. | • Verifies that services were provided and/or that clinical hours were earned. <br> • Schedules allow for time management and reminders of appointments. |

*(continues)*

**Figure 17-1** Clinical genres

| Clinical Reports | Description | Function |
|---|---|---|
| **Diagnostic Report** | When a client first comes to the clinic, his or her speech, language, and hearing are evaluated, and this document reports the evaluations. It could be written at any point in the semester, and is often cowritten, as students often work in a team to conduct testing. The parts of the report include *background information* (about the client's medical and speech therapy history), *types of tests conducted, description of each test, results from each test, summary of the results, clinical impressions* (the clinician's observations during testing), and *recommendations for therapy* based on the results. | ● Confirms or rules out communication disorders, differences, or delays, to determine the severity of the problem and to make recommendations for services. <br> ● Provides baseline data for planning treatment. |
| **Treatment Plan** | Written during the first few weeks of the semester, this document contains the following sections: *background information* (about the client's medical and speech therapy history), *goals* (for speech therapy), *rationales* (reasons for choosing the goals), *level of performance at beginning of semester* (to serve as a baseline), *objectives* (a breakdown of each goal), *program steps* (a breakdown of the steps that will be taken to achieve an objective), and approaches/procedures (a description of the treatment techniques the clinician will use). | ● Outlines the direction therapy will take that semester. <br> ● Is reviewed and signed by the student clinician, clinical supervisor, and client or client's guardian. |
| **Progress Report** | Written at the end of the semester, this document contains all the sections that the treatment plan used, but now includes results of each objective, summary of all the results, clinical impressions (observations made by the clinician and others who communicate regularly with the client), and recommendations (whether or not therapy should continue, what to focus on during the next semester, whether more evaluation should take place, whether the client should get support from other professionals, such as audiologists or occupational therapists). | ● Allows the clinician to review the progress with the client. <br> ● Provides a starting point for the next clinician. <br> ● Communicates results to multiple audiences. |

**Figure 17-1** (Continued)

# THE STAKES

Writing Across the Curriculum specialists talk about writing falling along a continuum of stakes, ranging from low stakes to high stakes, depending on the roles of the writing and the consequences or outcomes of the writing. Lesson plans may be considered lower stakes, as these documents have a limited audience and are not part of the client's permanent record. Daily notes and SOAP notes have slightly higher stakes, as they may be viewed by other professionals and insurance companies. Diagnostic and progress reports are considered high stakes writing, as these reports can determine how well a teacher or parent supports and supplements a child's program, how the next clinician follows up on the work you do this semester, and whether or not an insurance company covers expenses. The stakes are also, in part, determined by who the writer is. For example, though lesson plans may be considered lower stakes by experienced SLPs, the stakes go up when they are written by student clinicians. Lesson plans serve as a means of communication between the student clinician and clinical supervisor and are essential to the therapy process. Though experienced SLPs may write lesson plans as a matter of routine, beginning student clinicians may spend several hours developing effective plans for their clients before each session (Russell, 1995).

While the stakes can be high, there are ways to negotiate them. Each clinical report you compose may go through several drafts, and each draft presents an opportunity to receive feedback from your supervisor and other graduate students. This means that the pressure is off of the early drafts, although you always need to edit your work before submitting it to your clinical supervisor. You can use these drafts to take risks in your writing and try different ways of presenting and organizing information, and different ways of representing yourself and your client to multiple audiences. If deadlines limit your ability to follow these suggestions, you can still revise your work with a clinical supervisor or peers after you submitted the report to a client or professionals. You will then be more proficient the next time you need to produce a similar piece of writing.

# AUDIENCES

We often think of audience as singular—as one entity—but the audience for clinical writing, especially clinical reports, is multiple. Your audience could include the client, the client's family, teachers, other rehabilitation therapists, health care providers, insurance companies, or the legal system. The audience also includes your supervisors and, if the client continues therapy after this semester, the next speech-language clinician and other members of the team. One of the challenges of clinical writing is negotiating the needs and sensitivities of each potential audience member—communicating all that you want to say, while using a level of discourse that is specific enough for the professionals in the audience and accessible enough for the parents and some clients, who are less familiar with the terminology.

There are several strategies you can use to negotiate audience. One is a prewriting technique. Before writing a document, such as a progress report (a genre where balancing audiences becomes particularly tricky because so many audiences are involved), you can list the members of the audience, and then briefly freewrite (jot down notes) to each of these readers, saying exactly what you need this person to know. When you write the first draft of your report, refer to these freewrites to make sure you address all the points that you want to communicate.

Another technique is useful later in the writing process. Once you have a full draft, bring the draft to several readers who are similar to members of your audience. For instance, after removing identifying information, you could ask a person who is less familiar with CSD (such as a writing center consultant) to read the report to see if all of the language is accessible. You could ask a person who has considerable expertise with clinical writing (such as a clinical supervisor) to read the report to see if the language is specific enough. You could ask fellow graduate students to read it to see what picture they get of the client, and if they have a clear sense of how therapy would be continued next semester. These different sets of feedback can provide a fresh look at your writing through the eyes of your audience.

## READABILITY

Part of writing to an audience is making sure that the writing is reader-friendly. Readers gravitate to writing that feels warm and personal. However, the voice you use should also retain a professional tone. You want your reader to see you as both a caring therapist and a competent, knowledgeable professional whom they can trust. You can create this perception by using the word "I" to refer to yourself, a pronoun that is more personal than "the clinician," and shows confidence on the part of the writer. Using "I" also grammatically requires the active voice rather than the passive voice, a move that helps to close the gap between the reader and the text. For example, rather than saying that a test "was administered," you can simply say, "I administered the test." However, keep in mind that the word "I" may not be appropriate for all sections of a report, such as in behavioral objectives. In diagnostic reports, the word "we" may be more appropriate when a team of two or more clinicians is completing the evaluation. Also, keep in mind that there is controversy in the field about the use of "I." The American Psychological Association (APA) now endorses the use of first person pronouns in scientific writing. This has led to greater use in other forms of professional writing. We advise you to ask your on- and off-campus clinical supervisors about their perspective on this writing practice.

Creating a picture of who the client is as a person also makes clinical writing more reader-friendly. You can use the client's name in place of "the client" to make the writing sound more personal. In sections of clinical writing that are more narrative, such as the background information and clinical impressions, you can describe the client's interests and personality. Remember that the representation you create of your client will serve as the first impression of this client for the next clinician, so these pieces of information are doubly important. Keep in mind that the use of personal names and details varies from setting to setting. For example, in medical settings it is generally more common to refer to "the patient" in clinical writing as opposed to using proper names and there is less room for personal details.

Another part of readability is the way that writing looks on the page. The use of white space, bullets, tables, and paragraph length all affect the way a reader negotiates and decodes a text. You can enhance readability by breaking large chunks of prose into shorter paragraphs, using bullets to list information, and including tables to present quantitative information. Use these features to help a reader navigate your writing, and zone in on the important pieces of information. Be careful, though, not to sacrifice evaluative or interpretive statements in the name of conciseness. Lay readers rely on your interpretation of data; therefore, accompany your tables with explanations that help readers understand the data.

## "GOOD NEWS" AND "BAD NEWS"

Since student clinicians work closely with their clients and care about them, students sometimes have a difficult time delivering "bad news"—such as lack of progress, lack of an adequate support network for the client, or difficulty with a client's behavior during therapy. At UNH, we noticed this challenge during writing conferences. The clinical supervisor or writing fellow would finish reading a truly glowing progress report, and say to the student, "Wow—it sounds like everything went well." The student clinician would then talk about the not-so-good news. In addition, delivering "good news" in a progress report can be difficult. It is easy to become overly focused on the negatives and miss the small, but significant, increments of progress. These distortions of progress can result from being overly focused on a certain member of the audience, such as a young client's mother who has attended every therapy session, or the next clinician, who needs to be persuaded to follow the recommendations. The best strategy for making sure that the progress report reflects a client's progress is to conference with another student or clinical supervisor. Your reader could use a technique called "Say Back" (Elbow and Belanoff). After reading your progress report, readers share their overall impression from the report. You then have the opportunity to see if their impression matches what you wanted to convey. Your readers can also look to see if what you have reported in the various sections aligns with the recommendations. If the earlier sections are written in glowing terms, but are followed by an exhaustive list of recommendations (or if the opposite occurs), then a gap exists and you may want to consider revising.

# HANDLING BACKGROUND INFORMATION

Writing the background information section of the treatment plan and progress report can also be demanding. The challenge of writing this section was made apparent during a UNH practicum writing workshop. Students were asked to prepare for the workshop by analyzing the chart of one of their clients who had been coming to the clinic over a long period of time. During the workshop, several graduate students reported their surprise at the number of passages in recent documents that were copied word-for-word from earlier documents, particularly in the background information sections. This writing practice is not necessarily problematic in the way that other "copying" would be. Unlike other types of writing, clinical charts are collaboratively written, in that they are composed of writing by multiple authors. However, repeating passages from other clinical documents may not make the best impression on your readers, particularly those readers who have been reading reports from the clinic over a number of semesters. The background information section provides an opportunity to show your readers how well you know the client. To avoid repeating chunks of text verbatim from other reports, you could try a prewriting technique. After reading a chart, close it, put it away, and then jot down what you remember about the client. When writing the background information section, base your writing on these notes and only refer to the chart for specific information (i.e. doctors' names, dates).

This challenge of choosing what to omit when writing a background section is more applicable when the client has a thick chart (thus indicating that the client has been seen for services for a long time). While condensing the history for on-going clients has its own challenges, developing the history for a new client can be overwhelming. Rather than sorting through piles of information about the client, you are instead building a description from a variety of sources that may include a case history questionnaire, an initial interview, and referral forms. Once you write this description, you may need to step back and ask yourself if there are any gaps in your information. Do you need to know more about the client's medical condition? Do you understand why certain decisions were made by other professionals providing services? Do you have a clear sense of the client's communication ability? After writing a first draft of the background section, you may find yourself needing to ask the client and his or her team more questions and planning initial therapy sessions in such a way that will allow you to make additional observations to fill in any gaps.

# WRITING OBJECTIVES

Most forms of clinical writing reference goals and objectives either directly or indirectly. Setting treatment goals and writing specific objectives related to those goals form the crux of your clinical practice. Goals and objectives serve as a mutually agreed upon contract for the services you provide. They help you to narrow down and maintain your therapeutic focus. It is also important, however, to be mindful of the "big picture." In other words, you will need to regularly consider your client holistically in the context of a variety of his or her environments so that you do not lose sight of the broader communication skills and needs. For these reasons, it is especially important to formulate appropriate and reasonable objectives.

Your own developing philosophies about communication will be the guiding principles behind your intervention procedures. At times, you may feel that the objectives you develop may not directly reflect your personal hypotheses. It can be a challenge to reconcile a social/interactional view of communication intervention in situations where a behavioral objective format is required. One way to accomplish this is to provide a rationale for each objective. This can help a reader understand how the objective relates to the ultimate communication goal. Another way to accomplish this is to make sure that your focus is on improving the client's ability to communicate effectively in real-life situations, as opposed to simply correcting or reducing a problem. It may be reassuring for you to recognize that although the required objective *format* may be behavioral in nature, your overall *approach* to treatment can be based on a social-communicative perspective.

Objectives may take alternate forms in different practicum settings. In a school setting, the goals and objectives are generally connected to the curriculum. In a medical setting, the focus of objectives is typically on achieving functional, daily living outcomes. Do not hesitate to ask your supervisor how and why objectives may be written differently in each practicum experience you enter. In some cases, the objective may be fairly general—similar to a goal or benchmark, such as *"Sam will improve his conversational skills."* Other settings may require a more specific format, such as *"Sam will increase his ability to initiate conversations."* In other situations, you will need to develop a traditional behavioral objective that includes three components: skill/conditions/criteria, such as *"Sam will be able to initiate a conversation with familiar partners at least three times per day in response to an expectant gaze."* The traditional behavioral objective most clearly specifies what you expect an individual to achieve and is, therefore, useful as long as you keep sight of the ultimate communication goals. Now we turn to writing resources that you can seek to support your professional writing development.

# WRITING RESOURCES
• • • • • • • • • • • • • • • • • • • • • • • • • •

## Sample Clinical Documents

In each practicum setting you work in, ask if you can read samples of what your supervisor considers effective clinical documents for that setting (while maintaining confidentiality). Try to collect samples from the range of clinical genres used at that setting. In each setting, you can explore how that setting or situation shapes writing conventions, the implications of clinical writing for particular audiences, and how writing styles vary across individual clinicians. Your program may also keep copies of effectively written clinical reports from their on-campus or affiliated clinics. By skimming though these samples, you can get a sense of the range of styles and formats available to you. You can see the choices other student clinicians have made when deciding how to portray their voice, how much information to include, how to translate jargon for a lay audience, and how to negotiate the needs, concerns, and sensitivities of various members of the audience.

## Conferences with Supervisors

Your supervisors are important writing resources, as they provide a professional audience for your reports. Since your supervisors sign their names to your reports, they are mutually invested in both the treatment you give your clients and the way your reports are written. Conferences with your supervisors give you an opportunity to develop the writing skills you need both as a graduate student and as a professional in your field. To save time during the conference, give your supervisor an annotated draft ahead of time. On this draft, highlight areas you would like the supervisor to focus on and jot down any questions you have in the margins. These notes will show the supervisor how you view your own writing and where you are in the drafting process.

## Clinical Report Revision Guide

The Clinical Report Revision Guide, a resource developed collaboratively by CSD clinical faculty and Writing Across the Curriculum faculty at the University of New Hampshire is included in Figure 17-2. This guide is used by UNH clinical supervisors to help students reflect on their clinical writing. It is included here because we have found that when students complete the guide before meeting with clinical faculty, their clinical writing is stronger, discussion on writing during the meeting is more focused, and students need to revise their clinical writing less often. The revision guide can also be an important tool to use during the writing process as a way to check your own work. Feel free to adapt this form to fit the criteria in your program.

## Your Fellow Graduate Students

Your fellow graduate students can be your best writing resources. Plan to write in a computer cluster or student lounge at the same time, so that you can ask each other questions as you write. See if other students are interested in forming a writing group. Email drafts to each other to get advice. Set up times to meet to exchange drafts. These meetings can work as mini-deadlines to motivate you to get a draft completed early.

## Writing Resources at Your College or University

Writing centers, available at many colleges and universities, offer free one-on-one conferences with students on their writing. Writing center consultants can

**Name:** _____ **Date:** _____

Use this checklist as a guide for reviewing and editing your reports.

|  | Yes | No | Comments |
|---|---|---|---|
| As I was composing this report, I adjusted my writing with the intended audiences in mind by . . . |  |  |  |
| I used specialized/technical language when appropriate. When I did so, I provided brief definitions, examples, or context. |  |  |  |
| I reviewed this report to make sure that it is well-organized and chronologically accurate. |  |  |  |
| I eliminated unnecessary words and extraneous information. |  |  |  |
| I used simple sentences when appropriate. |  |  |  |
| I avoided excessive use of passive voice. |  |  |  |
| I used first-person pronouns (I, we) only when appropriate. |  |  |  |
| I proofread this report for spelling, grammar, and punctuation. |  |  |  |

*(continues)*

**Figure 17-2** UNH Clinical Report Revision Guide (front)

| | Yes | No | Comments |
|---|---|---|---|
| I included phonetic symbols if needed. | | | |
| I shared this report with another person for feedback (while maintaining confidontiality) and discovered . . . | | | |
| I read this report aloud and noticed . . . | | | |
| I have adjusted identifying information and background sections to reflect any changes since the treatment plan by . . . | | | |
| I have adjusted the verb tense of each section as needed. | | | |

Which part of the report was easiest to write?  Why?

_____

_____

_____

Which part of the report was the most challenging to write?  Why?

_____

_____

_____

If I had more time, I would change/revise . . .

_____

_____

_____

**Figure 17-2** UNH Clinical Report Revision Guide (back)

offer you the perspective of a lay reader, a perspective that neither your clinical supervisor nor a fellow graduate student can offer. You may find this perspective particularly helpful when composing clinical reports, as opposed to clinical documentation. Remember to remove identifying information from documents before visiting the writing center. Writing centers also usually have writing guides and computer clusters available to students.

## Report Forms and Templates

Many programs provide their students with some sort of guide for writing clinical reports, such as treatment plans and progress reports. These guides range from skeletal outlines of a report's organization to more elaborately detailed descriptions of what information could be included in each section of a report. If these guides are available electronically, they can provide you with re-usable formats for tables and examples of test descriptions that are easily understandable to a lay audience. While these guides can be helpful, they can also be misleading, in that they imply that clinical writing is a simple process of filling in the blanks. Also, these guides can imply that clinical genres are inflexible—that the specifications of each section are set in stone. Be sure to ask your clinical supervisor questions about how each clinical genre can be adapted to fit the demands of specific writing situations.

## Writing Guides

There are several writing guides available that focus on professional writing in CSD, such as *Report Writing for Speech-Language Pathologists and Audiologists*, 2nd Edition by Pannbacker, Middleton, Vekovius, & Sanders, (2001); *Survival Guide for the Beginning Speech-Language Clinician* by Moon-Meyer, (1998); *Report Writing in the Field of Communication Disorders: A Handbook for Students and Clinicians, 2nd Edition,* by Knepflar and May, (1992); and *A Coursebook on Scientific & Professional Writing for Speech-Language Pathology, 3rd Edition,* by Hegde (2003). These guides provide writing techniques, sample reports, and grammar lessons.

## CONCLUSION

It is important to keep in mind that you will not learn everything about clinical writing during your graduate program. Learning professional writing is a lifelong process, as are many aspects of our professional work. It is this continual learning process that makes our role as therapists so satisfying. Throughout our career, we continue to develop expertise as we face new challenges, meet new clients, write in new genres, and are introduced to new ideas about human interaction and communication. As an integral part of client care, clinical writing makes a real difference in people's lives.

## WORKS CITED

American Psychological Association. (2001). *Publication manual of the American Psychological Association* (5th ed.). Washington, DC: Author.

Elbow, P. & Belanoff, P. (2000). *Sharing and responding* (3rd ed.). Boston: McGraw-Hill.

Hegde, M.N. (2003). *A coursebook on scientific & professional writing for speech-language pathology* (3rd ed.). Clifton Park, NY: Thomson Delmar Learning

Knepflar, K. & May, E. (1992). *Report writing in the field of communication disorders.* (2nd ed.). Rockville, MD: ASHA Publications.

Meyer, S.M. (1998). *Survival guide for the beginning speech-language clinician.* Gaithersburg, MD: Aspen Publishers, Inc.

Pannbacker, M., Middleton, G., Vekovius, G., & Sanders, K. (2001). *Report writing for speech-language pathologists and audiologists.* (2nd ed.). Austin, TX: Pro ed.

Russell, D. *"Activity theory and its implications for writing instruction." Reconceiving writing: Rethinking writing instruction.* Ed. J. Petraglia. Mahwah, NJ: Erlbaum (1995). 51–77.

# CHAPTER 18

## Advice for First-Year Graduate Students

### INTRODUCTION

You have made it to graduate school! You are now working towards earning a master's or doctorate, depending on your personal goals. The next two to five years will be very challenging, but they will also be rewarding. Remind yourself why you are going through the obstacles, and be grateful for the opportunities to take on the challenges. Remember that there is a light at the end of the tunnel. You will not be in graduate school forever. Before you know it, you will be working with individuals with communication disorders and their families. You will soon be making a positive impact on their quality of life. This chapter provides some tips for succeeding in graduate school and Figure 18-1 can be used as a checklist to track your progress.

## Make the Most of Graduate School

You will not have another time in your life when you will have faculty members at your fingertips to teach you and answer your questions. Right now, if you have almost any question related to a client, you are just a phone call, email, or appointment away from problem solving with a professor or clinical instructor. You may not have this same kind of support once you are professionally practicing. Take advantage of all that your professors have to teach you!

## Make an Effort at the Beginning of the Semester to Meet Each of Your Peers

Your classmates will become one of your most valuable resources. You never know when you will need to call a classmate to discuss, or vent about, a challenging class. By making a concerted effort to meet students in your classes at the beginning of each semester, you will be building a wide network of support. Consider inviting classmates out for coffee to discuss a class, experiences, the graduate program, or other common interests. Establish a way of contacting fellow students by phone and/or email. Form study groups and work on assignments when your professor allows it. The relationships you form with your peers in graduate school can lead to professional alliances years down the road.

☐ Make the most of graduate school.

☐ Make an effort at the beginning of the semester to meet each of your peers.

☐ Make friends inside and outside of the department.

☐ If you want a roommate, consider one from your department.

☐ Make time for yourself.

☐ Have good self-care.

☐ If you think you might have a mental health condition, seek professional help.

☐ Find a second-year graduate student to be your mentor.

☐ Organize graduation-related papers in a binder.

☐ Make a timeline of your courses from now until graduation.

☐ Purchase a large backpack, briefcase, or rolling computer bag with a handle.

☐ Take breaks while studying to keep yourself alert.

☐ Do your best without being too hard on yourself.

☐ Learn to do things efficiently.

☐ Balance your coursework and clinical work.

☐ When you do not have time to read chapters and/or articles, skim them before class.

☐ Try to complete assignments early.

☐ Use your professors' office hours and email addresses.

☐ Be open with professors and clinical instructors when you are over-whelmed.

☐ Save all of your notes, handouts, and books.

☐ Take things one hour at a time.

☐ Make daily and/or weekly lists of tasks to complete.

☐ Take advantage of the educational opportunities offered.

**Figure 18-1** Checklist for first-year graduate students

# Make Friends Inside and Outside of the Department

Forming a strong support group of friends will make graduate school much easier and more enjoyable. Meet friends outside of your department by joining a club, volunteer organization, or honor society; taking an interdisciplinary class; attending a place of worship that has activities for young adults and/or graduate students; or joining a sports team. Also, make time to call or visit family. Graduate school is important, but so is spending time with friends and family.

# If You Want a Roommate, Consider One from Your Department

A roommate from the department is great for working on assignments, reminding each other about due dates, quizzing each other, carpooling, relating to each other's experiences, and encouraging each other. If you are transferring to a new school, ask the secretary if she or he is allowed to email all of the new graduate students to find out if anyone needs a roommate, or if there is a bulletin board in the department where you can post roommate-wanted flyers. Some students prefer to have roommates outside of their department. Other students prefer to live on their own because they do not feel comfortable living with someone they do not know (e.g., if they are a first-year student in a new city), have had too many negative experiences with roommates, or a number of other reasons. Try to find a living situation where you will be most comfortable because not only are you likely to spend time there working on coursework, but it is also nice to get away from school and go "home" to relax.

# Make Time for Yourself

You may get so busy that you forget to take time for yourself. Make time to do things for yourself, even if it is just for 10 minutes. Reward yourself by doing the little things that make life enjoyable, such as listening to your favorite CD on the way to class, reading a novel on the bus ride home from class, making your favorite dinner, packing your favorite snack in your lunch, watching your favorite television show in the evening, going to a jazz concert, taking a yoga class, learning how to swing dance, attending a prayer group, going to a basketball game, joining a frisbee club, taking a pottery class, going to a Karaoke club with friends, visiting your family, or hanging out with your siblings or cousins. The possibilities are endless! Do whatever you can to help maintain your peace of mind and keep your stress levels in check during graduate school. Things will get tough, and you need something to look forward to each week.

# Have Good Self-Care

It may seem like common sense, but when graduate school gets hectic, you might be surprised how easy it can be to forget to take care of yourself. Get enough sleep, eat three healthy meals per day, work out at least a few times per week, and drink plenty of water to stay hydrated. Always have a water bottle with you. When you take care of yourself, it should be easier to do your work and get the most out of your graduate experience.

If your department's building has a locker, refrigerator, and/or microwave that graduate students can use, always store some extra food like canned fruit, pretzels, or soup in your locker. You never know when you will have to spend an unexpected five hours working on a project in your department's building. If your department does not have a refrigerator and microwave for students, petition to get them. Suggest that your NSSLHA chapter do fundraisers and ask the department chair if the department can match funds.

If you are mostly off-campus for externships, always have some extra food in the trunk of your car or in your backpack. If you drive, you may also want to keep an extra pair of workout clothes in your trunk in case you end up having fifteen to thirty extra minutes to go to a local gym, or go for a run or walk outside on a nice day.

# If You Think You Might Have a Mental Health Condition, Seek Professional Help

It is not uncommon for students in graduate school (regardless of discipline) to go through a period of depression. If you find yourself feeling depressed, experiencing anxiety, developing an eating disorder, not being able to sleep or any other mental health condition, seek professional help right away. Similarly, if you have a friend who appears to have a mental health condition, encourage him or her to seek help. Most campuses have mental health offices where you can speak with a counselor confidentially. Also consider seeking help from a priest, parent, mentor, and/or close friend. However, if you or a friend ever have suicidal thoughts, it is essential to seek help from a medical professional at a hospital. Many campuses also have a mental health crisis hotline. Search your university's Web site to find out the number and do not be afraid to use it no matter how late at night it may be.

If you are diagnosed with a mental health issue, you may want to alert your professors to your condition if it is negatively affecting your performance. However, this is your private health information, so you are not required to disclose it. Realize that most academic programs understand about these sorts of issues. In severe mental health conditions, you and your doctor/family may decide that it is best for you to take time off from school. In this case, contact your department chair and request a leave of absence. Then, you can resume your program when you are better.

# Find a Second-Year Graduate Student to Be Your Mentor

To help you acclimate to the graduate program, the school, or the location, consider asking a second-year graduate student to be a mentor. Some graduate programs have a buddy system that is organized through the NSSLHA chapter. It is always easier to get through coursework when your peers are there for emotional and academic support. If there is no such program, consider starting one.

# Organize Graduation-Related Papers in a Binder

At the beginning of your program, you may receive information about courses, teaching certification, ASHA certification, portfolio requirements, and thesis and/or dissertation requirements. You are likely to forget about the information once classes begin, but professors and classmates will occasionally mention the important information throughout your program. Having these papers in a special binder will make it easy for you to access the information when you have questions.

# Make a Timeline of Your Courses from Now until Graduation and Put It into Your Binder

You probably received a list of courses that you are required to take at the beginning of your program. In addition you should have some electives you can choose. Often, graduate courses are only offered once per academic year. Thus, it is a good idea to plan early in your first year for courses you need/want to take during the next few years. This will increase your chances of taking the elective courses that interest you the most.

If you went to an undergraduate institution that is different from your graduate institution, you should make an appointment with your academic advisor to determine whether you are missing any courses. If you are lucky, you may find that you do not have to take one or two courses because you had them as an undergraduate.

# Purchase a Large Backpack, Briefcase, or Rolling Computer Bag with a Handle

As a graduate student, you will have a lot of materials to carry with you. A normal sized backpack may not be large enough. You will have many binders and textbooks to bring with you to class, especially on days when you have more than one class and a client. You may want to consider a backpack with wheels and a handle, an extra large backpack, or even a rolling computer bag with a handle.

## Take Breaks While Studying to Keep Yourself Alert

You may find yourself buried underneath all the studying necessary to get through your classes. For many people, breaks are needed to keep your mind (and body) alert. If you are tired or your brain starts "zoning," you are no longer getting the most out of your efforts. If you are at home, you could do your laundry or housework between assignments. If you are on campus or in the library, consider taking a 15-minute walk to clear your mind, or consider changing locations. Spend a few hours studying in the library, then move to a coffee house for a change of scenery.

## Do Your Best without Being Too Hard on Yourself

Know that you probably do not have the time to give everything 110% like you may have as an undergraduate. Those of you who are perfectionists may have to let go of some of your perfectionist tendencies when you work on assignments. Otherwise, you will not get all of your work done because there simply is not enough time in a day or week. Also, realize that it is not life or death—it's just graduate school!

## Learn To Do Things Efficiently

You will find that much of graduate school is learning how to do things efficiently within a small amount of time. Your time management skills will be challenged daily. Learning to complete tasks efficiently is a skill that you will use throughout the rest of your life as a clinician, doctoral student, researcher, spouse, parent, or whatever roles you have. Refer to Appendix A for some tools that might help you stay organized to get things done efficiently.

## Balance Your Coursework and Clinical Work

Balancing coursework and clinical work are both important to being a good clinician. Students may fall into a routine of spending most of their time on clinical work, but neglecting their traditional courses. Designate time to read your textbooks, work on assignments, and prepare for clinical practica. Try to get into a routine early in the semester.

## When You Do Not Have Time to Read Chapters and/or Articles, Skim Them Before Class

While ideally you will always completely read assignments before class, in reality this may not always be possible. If you can not read chapters or articles ahead of time, skim them before class so that you are familiar with the concepts. If a chapter has chapter objectives, take a few minutes to familiarize yourself with them. Then you can quickly refer to your books and/or articles in the future when you are searching for specific information. If you were an undergraduate who had time to read all of your chapters/articles before class, you may find it frustrating that you do not have enough time to read all of the assigned readings in graduate school.

## Try to Complete Assignments Early

When you have a week where you do not have a lot of assignments due, get ahead for the following week. You will find that assignments are a lot easier to complete when you are not working under the stress of getting them done the day before—or sometimes the same day—they are due. Plus, if you have questions on your assignments, you will have time to ask your professor. Using a lighter week to get ahead may mean keeping what could have been a really stressful, hectic week, more manageable.

## Use Your Professors' Office Hours and Email Addresses

Advice regarding professor's office hours is the same regardless of whether you are a freshman in college or a graduate student; take advantage of office hours. Meet with your professor if you do not understand something. Do not be afraid to email your professor or stay after class and seek help if you need it. You are paying your professors to teach you the concepts and answer your questions. Get your money's worth! Besides, most professors enjoy students who are inquisitive and want to learn more about a topic.

## Be Open with Professors and Clinical Instructors When You Are Overwhelmed

If you are overwhelmed by your coursework, be open with your professors. Let them know that you are trying hard. They may be expecting too much. They may change an aspect of the course if they realize that they have unrealistic expectations. If you are overwhelmed in part because of personal reasons outside of class, such as a death in the family or an illness, let your professors and clinical instructors know. They will probably be willing to provide you with extra support, or possibly let you take an incomplete grade if things are too overwhelming. As mentioned earlier, you may want to seek counseling services on campus to help you through difficult times.

## Save All of Your Notes, Handouts, and Books

Notes, handouts, and books will be valuable resources when you are an independent clinician and/or researcher. They will also help if you take the Praxis, a comprehensive exam needed to work in some states and for ASHA certification. Set up a system for filing and storing these materials so you can easily access them if needed for another class, a clinical experience, or studying for the Praxis.

## Take Things One Hour at a Time

Literally say to yourself, "what do I want to concentrate on for the next hour?" Sometimes, you just need to take a deep breath and do what you can. If you look at all the things to be accomplished during a week, it can get overwhelming. Focus on accomplishing things in smaller increments and you may feel more successful and less stressed.

## Make Daily and/or Weekly Lists of Tasks to Complete

Do not tell yourself you have too much to do and there is no time to make a list. Take five minutes to write down what you need to get done that day or that week. Prioritize based upon what is due first—complete a reading assignment, go online for an article, email a professor, etc—and depending on how you work, update the list as you need to keep on track. You may want to have a list of what goals you want to accomplish by the end of the year. Making a list and using it to keep organized is a good way to prevent those late night worries from keeping you up. If you find yourself having a hard time falling asleep because you are worrying about all the things you need to accomplish, get up, make a list, and try to go back to sleep. You might be surprised by how much more at ease your mind is (and how much easier sleep comes).

## Take Advantage of the Educational Opportunities Offered

Your department and university may offer a wide range of additional educational opportunities. Check your university and department calendars for educational opportunities, such as seminars, that interest you. Take advantage of continuing education courses to fine tune your skills. Computer, literature search, and writing courses may be available through your university or a local community college. These courses often meet once for a few hours. Graduate school is a wonderful time to gather information you will use everyday when you are a clinician and/or researcher. Make the most of your time in graduate school.

## CONCLUSION

There are many characteristics that make for a successful graduate student. As you can see from the tips discussed in this chapter, organization is key. Figure 18-2 lists some additional characteristics that are important. Knowing and developing these characteristics can help you get the most out of your first year as a graduate student.

Want to know if you have what it takes to be a clinician? See how well you match up with these attributes.

- *Dedication.* Your program of study is intensive and extensive.

- *Flexibility.* You need to have the ability to work with a variety of people in a variety of settings.

- *Teachability.* You must be willing to learn from others with different approaches and views.

- *Compassion.* This is a service-oriented profession. You need to demonstrate a caring attitude to those served.

- *Reliability.* Those served must be able to depend on your presence as well as your knowledge.

- *Persistence.* Keep working to find the best possible solution.

- *Curiosity.* Keep investigating causes and concerns.

- *Accountability.* Document your work and keep records.

- *Ethics.* You will address confidential issues on a daily basis. The clients, supervisors, and future employers must be able to rely on your ethical behavior.

- *Appropriate behavior.* Develop the ability to interact with others in an appropriately professional manner. This includes your conversation and your appearance.

- *Academic proficiency.* Trying to maintain a balance is difficult, but you must maintain adequate academic proficiency.

- *A sense of humor!*

**Figure 18-2** Characteristics of successful graduate clinicians

# CHAPTER 19

# Advice for Second-Year Graduate Students

## INTRODUCTION

As a master's student, you may be planning to enter the workforce at the completion of your degree. After all your years of schooling and training, you are getting closer to your career as an audiologist, speech-language pathologist, or speech, language, and hearing scientist. There are a number of things to accomplish during your master's program and this chapter provides advice for successfully reaching graduation. Figure 19-1 is a checklist for you to use to track your progress. When beginning your master's program, you may be undecided about whether to pursue a doctorate. You do not need this planned out in your first year of your master's program, but you should be prepared to make a decision by your second year, as you will need to go through the application process to enter a doctoral program. Remember, as an SLP, you can enter the workforce for a few years to gain experience before applying to doctoral programs.

## Follow Your Clinical Instructor's Suggestions and Timelines

Your clinical instructor provides instruction and guidance to help you become a good clinician. If you do not see why it would be beneficial to do things the way that the clinical instructor suggests, ask him or her to explain more about it. At least try what the clinical instructor suggests; you may be surprised how well most suggestions work. Clinical instructors usually like to see students incorporating their suggestions into sessions.

## Identify a Mentor If You Do Not Already Have One

A mentor is an experienced professional you can contact for guidance and information. This person can be a professor, clinical instructor, doctoral student, or clinician who is willing to let you ask questions. A mentor is also a person who you can look up to and strive to be like. Your master's program may have

☐ Follow your clinical instructor's suggestions and timelines.

☐ Identify a mentor if you do not already have one.

☐ Learn about state certification and ASHA certification.

☐ If you are interested in research, inquire about research assistantships or hourly rate positions.

☐ Seek other assistantship positions.

☐ Consider writing a thesis.

☐ Become active with your local chapter of NSSLHA.

☐ Join NSSLHA.

☐ Join an ASHA Special Interest Division.

☐ Attend the ASHA Convention, state convention, and other related conferences.

☐ Participate in a poster session during the ASHA convention.

☐ Request clinical instructors or supervisors who specialize in an area that interests you.

☐ Keep your options open about areas of specialization.

☐ Identify your strengths and weaknesses.

☐ Create a portfolio.

☐ Prepare for the Comprehensive Exams.

☐ Start looking for an externship position.

☐ If you want to work in a school setting, make sure you know the requirements.

☐ Start preparing for the Praxis.

☐ Identify a clinical fellowship position at the beginning of your last semester of graduate school.

☐ Consider doctoral study.

☐ Take the Praxis during your last semester of graduate study.

☐ Apply for state certification and/or licensure after graduation.

☐ Convert your membership from NSSLHA to ASHA.

**Figure 19-1** Advice for second-year graduate students

a mentorship program in place. If it does, take advantage of it. If not, ASHA has several programs that will match students with mentors. Visit the Student Section of the ASHA Web site for more detailed information about these resources. Mentors are key in succeeding in CSD, and you may find you have mentors well into clinical practice.

## Learn About State Certification and ASHA Certification

Ask your academic advisor, mentor, or clinic instructor about state and ASHA certification requirements. Make a timeline of what you need to do during your graduate program to be eligible for certification when you graduate. Ensure that your knowledge and skills acquisition (KASA) summaries are kept up to date and filled out correctly. Now that you are moving towards being a professional, it is important to take responsibility for knowing these requirements and following whatever steps are needed to obtain them.

## If You Are Interested in Research, Inquire About Research Assistantships or Hourly Rate Positions

If you are interested in learning more about research, identify a professor in your department who is conducting research that interests you. Since most schools have a limited number of assistantships, apply early if there is more than one deadline. Assistantship opportunities may vary throughout the year, as can the compensation for participation. For instance, a professor may look for a research assistant after receiving a grant during the middle of an academic year. Depending on the level of research needed, there can be a wide range of methods for compensating you for your time and effort. Keep your eyes and ears open throughout the year for assistantships. Be an advocate for yourself because professors are unlikely to seek you out to give you a job.

If assistantships are unavailable, ask about working for a professor at an hourly rate, such as a work-study. Sometimes you can volunteer and earn academic credit. Working for a professor will allow the professor to get to know you. If and when the professor has an assistantship position available, he or she will be more likely to hire someone he or she knows. Furthermore, working with a professor, regardless of the position, will be a valuable learning experience.

## Seek Other Assistantship Positions

There are assistantship programs beyond research assistant that can be valuable learning experiences and can help offset the cost of your education. These opportunities include teaching, clinical, and project assistantships. Ask your advisor for more information. You can also look on your department's Web site, and on department Web sites in related fields, such as psychology, communications, laryngeal physiology, and special education for these opportunities.

## Consider Writing a Thesis

Do you enjoy research? Do you like to ask questions and try to solve them? Talk with your mentor, advisor, and other students who have written a thesis. Ask about the process and the advantages and disadvantages. Different master's programs approach the thesis differently. If you are interested, find out if writing a thesis may prolong your graduation date, if any extra courses are required, and how much time per week most students spend on a thesis. Chapters 15 and 16 provide more information on the basics of research and writing a thesis.

## Become Active with Your Local Chapter of NSSLHA

See Chapter 3 for more information on NSSLHA. As a master's student, you can benefit greatly from membership in NSSLHA. Many events organized by the chapter will provide you with the opportunity for academic, professional, and social growth. If your program's chapter is primarily undergraduate, make the initiative to contact the NSSLHA chapter advisor and president to have chapter membership and events for graduate students. Suggest to the advisor and president the creation of a graduate student liaison position and offer to spearhead this or run for an officer position. Encourage your classmates to come to meetings and events.

If your program does not have a local chapter of NSSLHA, then start one at your university. Information for starting a local chapter is available on the NSSLHA Web site.

## Join NSSLHA

Graduate students who maintain two consecutive years of membership in NSSLHA at the time of graduation from a master's program are eligible to receive a significant discount off the initial membership and certification fees for ASHA. If you have not joined NSSLHA at any other point in your academic career, now is the time. Refer to Chapter 3 for more information on how to apply for national membership.

## Join an ASHA Special Interest Division

As you are getting further into your graduate studies, you may have some specific interests that are guiding your studies. Start interacting with other individuals who share similar special interests. ASHA recognizes different divisions where members can affiliate with a network of professionals and students with similar interests. Refer to Chapter 32 for more information.

## Attend the ASHA Convention, State Convention, and Other Related Conferences

Chapters 7, 8, 9, and 10 encouraged you to attend conventions and conferences during your undergraduate studies. As a master's student, attending these events will become even more important to your academic and professional development. More information about the benefits of attending the annual ASHA convention is available in Chapter 30.

## Participate in a Poster Session During the ASHA Convention

ASHA usually announces the Call for Papers (CFP) in January with an April deadline. Announcements will appear in the *ASHA Leader* and on the ASHA and NSSLHA Web sites. This is your opportunity to share your research with a captive audience. Take advantage of this platform and present what you have been working on at a poster session.

## Request Clinical Instructors or Supervisors Who Specialize in an Area That Interests You

If you have a specialty area that particularly interests you, ask the clinic director if students are allowed to request clinical instructors or supervisors who share your interest. This can be a great way to hone in on your area of interest and gain invaluable experience working in the specialty. See Chapter 25 for special interests in audiology and hearing sciences and Chapter 26 for specialty interests in speech-language pathology and speech-language sciences.

## Keep Your Options Open About Areas of Specialization

You may have a driving interest in a single area of specialization, such as adults versus children, medical versus school setting, and more specific areas, such as cochlear implants, craniofacial anomolies, or stroke. Do not lock yourself into one specialty interest. Take advantage of opportunities to learn about all aspects of the field. You may find an area that you love that you would have never considered before taking a course on it. Many students go into their graduate program set on working with children instead of adults. However, by the end of the program, they only want to work with adults. Even if there is an area that you swear you will never go into, take a seminar or attend a workshop at a convention on it. Plus, you never know when you will need to know about a specialty area. Stay open!

## Identify Your Strengths and Weaknesses

While you are in graduate school and have clinical instructors available to assist you in becoming a better clinician, identify your strengths and weaknesses. By recognizing your strengths and weaknesses while still in graduate school, you will have more support both in addressing the weaknesses and in highlighting the strengths. If you have a choice of practica, choose at least one practicum that you know the least about. It will be easier to improve your skills while in a graduate program than when you are a practicing clinician.

## Create a Portfolio

Having a portfolio when interviewing can be a tool that makes you stand apart from other applicants. Some employers, particularly schools, require a portfolio for an interview. Portfolios generally include written samples of your paperwork from different clinical settings, types of disorders you have worked with, examples of diagnostic and treatment tools used, state and national conferences you attended, national examinations you have passed, your resumé, and other relevant information. Some graduate programs require electronic portfolios, whereas other programs require paper portfolios. Ask your clinic director or an advisor about what specific information you should include.

## Prepare for the Comprehensive Exams

Some programs require master's students to take comprehensive exams (comps) prior to graduation. The comps are an exam that is given after the first year or during the last year of a master's program to assess what students have learned. However, other programs use the Praxis instead of comps. Ask your advisor or the department chairperson if your program has comprehensive exams and when they are offered. Find out if your program hosts meetings or reviews throughout the year to prepare for the comps. Attend these meetings and start studying early. Studying for both the comps and Praxis around the same time is helpful because studying for one will prepare you for the other.

# Start Looking for an Externship Position

If your program does not assign externship positions, start looking for one independently. Externship positions are community placements where you complete your graduate clinical experiences under direct supervision of an ASHA-certified audiologist or speech-language pathologist (if you are seeking ASHA certification). In many programs, externships occur during one or two semesters, usually during your second or third year of study. However, a few graduate programs do not have a department clinic and may have you do an externship during your first semester. Contact your department's clinic director/coordinator to find out who is responsible for arranging externship positions.

If you have to find externship positions on your own, there are several options to consider. If you have previous volunteer experience in a clinic, hospital, or school where audiology or speech-language pathology services are offered, these locations may be more receptive to taking you on as an extern. However, do not feel limited by your past experiences. You should seek out novel opportunities and consider contacting other places that you believe could offer beneficial experiences. As you seek out externships, remember that your supervisor must hold ASHA's Certificate of Clinical Competence (CCC) if you are seeking ASHA certification.

# If You Want to Work in a School Setting, Make Sure You Know the Requirements

Most states require professionals to take a certain number of education and special education courses and have teaching experience. Some states may require an exam related to special education. For instance, the exam may ask about the Individuals with Disabilities Education Act (IDEA). Consult with your advisor, state board of education, and/or an audiologist/speech-language pathologist who currently works in schools for more details regarding individual state requirements. Remember that it is your responsibility to seek out and comply with the requirements.

# Start Preparing for the Praxis

The Praxis is an exam designed by the Education Testing Service (ETS) to assess the competency of audiologists and speech-language pathologists as they enter their respective fields. The exam is sometimes called "the ASHA Exam," "the ASHA Boards," or "NESPA" (this is an older term that is rarely used anymore). Audiology students must take the audiology version of the exam, and speech-language pathology students must take the speech-language pathology version. The exams cover material taught during undergraduate and graduate courses.

To become an ASHA-certified audiologist or speech-language pathologist, students must score 600 or higher on the Praxis II. Most states require the same score for certification; however, some employers are only interested in scores higher than 600, such as 650 or 700. The exam can be repeated and does not average scores. ASHA does not offer a Praxis prep course; however, resources for preparing for the Praxis are available in the Student section of the ASHA Web site at http://www.asha.org. Start studying for the Praxis exam early in your final year of your master's program.

If you are applying for ASHA Certification, you are required to have a copy of your Praxis report mailed to ASHA. As part of a graduation requirement, your graduate program may require a report of your scores as well. Ask your advisor if the department needs your scores.

## Identify a Clinical Fellowship Position at the Beginning of Your Last Semester of Graduate School

In order to be ASHA certified in speech-language pathology, you need to complete a clinical fellowship (CF) after you graduate. The CF lays the foundation for the rest of your professional career. Take your time identifying a supervisor who is best able to provide you with support and encouragement through this period. More importantly, make sure that this individual is ASHA certified. It is during this time that you will be working and gaining the professional experience that you need in order to receive your Certificate of Clinical Competence (CCC).

## Consider Doctoral Study

Why stop at the master's level? Expand your employability and career options by obtaining a doctoral degree. Talk with your advisor about this degree and stop by the Graduate School Fair at the ASHA Convention. Many doctoral programs offer significant scholarships and financial aid. Additionally, the job market looks extremely bright for individuals with a Ph.D. working in a university setting. If you are interested in research and/or teaching, you should consider a doctorate degree. Detailed information regarding degree requirements is available on the Membership and Certification pages of the ASHA Web site.

A list of ASHA-accredited doctoral programs is available in Appendix B of this guide.

## Take the Praxis During Your Last Semester of Graduate Study

Many students chose to take this exam during their last semester of master's study, you can choose to take the exam earlier. Taking the exam earlier can relieve some anxiety because you know you will have a chance to take the exam again and prepare for the areas where you are weakest. Go to the Teaching and Learning Division of the Praxis Web site at http://www. teachingandlearning.org to find out more about registering for the exam.

## Apply for State Certification and/or Licensure After Graduation

Once you have successfully completed the Praxis Exam, your passing scores should be sent to the professional boards of your state for you to obtain state certification or licensure. Realize that every state has different requirements for submitting the scores. Research your state's requirements for certification on the state association page of the ASHA Web site. Remember that it is your responsibility to know what type of certification or licensure is needed for the type of setting in which you will work. Do not assume that your employer will tell you what certification or licensure is required.

## Convert Your Membership from NSSLHA to ASHA

Students who maintain two consecutive years of NSSLHA membership qualify for the NSSLHA-to-ASHA Conversion Discount Program. This discount provides a savings on the initial fees for membership and certification in ASHA. A significant number of students lose eligibility for the discount every year because they wait until the last minute to convert their membership. You do not have to wait until you complete your CF to apply to ASHA. You simply need to submit your application by August 31 of the year following graduation to apply at the reduced rate. If you are not sure whether you qualify for the Conversion Program Discount or when you need to convert your membership, contact the NSSLHA office at nsslha@asha.org before your master's graduation date.

## CONCLUSION

Depending on your course of study and your career goals (audiology versus speech-language pathology), your master's program may be the final degree you will need before beginning to practice professionally, or it may be one more step toward acquiring your doctoral degree. This chapter provides excellent advice for keeping track of the many things to be accomplished as a second-year graduate student. The checklist in Figure 19-1 can be a useful tool in tracking your progress. If you have obtained your master's, passed the Praxis, obtained certification, and are ready to enter the job force, congratulations! You have made significant achievements during your CSD studies and are about to embark on an incredible journey that will positively impact the quality of life for many people with communication disorders.

If you are preparing to enter a doctoral program to continue your studies, congratulations to you as well! Your educational journey will continue to provide you with exciting new academic, research, and clinical experiences, which will help shape the future contributions you make to the field.

# Doctoral Degrees and Applying to a Doctoral Program

Larissa Fedak, NSSLHA Regional Councilor, Region II, 2002–2004;
Marie Patton, master's student, SLP, University of Wisconsin-
Madison and NSSLHA President, 2001-2003; and Jeremy
Federman, NSSLHA Regional Councilor, Region III, 2003–2005

## INTRODUCTION

Chapter 2 provided an overview of the job outlook and salaries for audiologist and SLPs. The most striking data reported consisted of the positive job outlook for individuals with a doctorate. There is a misperception that a career in CSD is not advantageous; in truth, a career in CSD can be very rewarding for those with a doctorate degree. It is important for students to get a better understanding of doctoral study. The profession is facing a critical shortage of professionals with advanced degrees and is in serious need of a 'next generation' of individuals with these qualifications. This chapter provides an overview of the types of doctoral degrees in the United States and how to apply to a doctoral program. The rewards of obtaining a doctoral degree and the professional opportunities this opens up are immense, and you are strongly encouraged to investigate this possibility further.

## TYPES OF DEGREES IN THE UNITED STATES

Doctorates in CSD are typically oriented in one of two directions, clinical or research. Students who opt for a clinical doctorate often spend most of their career practicing clinically or working directly with clients assessing and providing treatment. In contrast, students who decide on a research doctorate will spend most of their career conducting research and teaching in hearing, speech, and language sciences.

The following are the most common doctoral degree designators available for students in CSD:

- Ph.D., Doctorate of Philosophy (clinical and/or research)
- Au.D., Doctorate of Audiology (clinical)

- Sc.D., Doctorate of Science (clinical and/or research)
- SLPD, Doctorate of Speech-Language Pathology (clinical)
- Ed.D., Doctorate of Education (clinical and/or research)

## APPLYING TO A DOCTORAL PROGRAM

The application process for clinical doctorates (e.g., Au.D.) is similar to applying to a master's program. The following general information will help students specifically interested in obtaining a doctoral degree in research (e.g., Ph.D.) apply to a program. If you are interested in the Sc.D., SLPD, or Ed.D., many of the steps are similar, but contact the programs you are specifically interested in for any requirements beyond what is covered here.

### Make Sure You Understand Why You Want to Pursue a Doctorate Degree

When you are applying to the program, be prepared to discuss why you want to pursue a doctorate degree beyond wanting to make money. The answers to this question, as well as your individual story explaining how and why you have become interested in taking this next step in your educational career, will largely determine if you will get accepted to a program. Furthermore, your reasons for pursing this degree are important for staying motivated enough to finish the program. These questions are but a small sample of potential questions you may be asked when applying to programs:

- Are you interested in basic or clinical research?
- What academic, clinical, and research experiences do you have, if any?
- What topics do you want to investigate?
- Do you want to be a professor?
- What teaching experiences have you had, if any?

### Do Not Rule Out a Ph.D. in a Related Field

After reflecting on your interests, you may realize you need to pursue a Ph.D. in a related field instead (e.g., education, family science, neurology, epidemiology, engineering), or in an interdisciplinary setting (e.g., cognitive science, rehabilitative sciences, child development). Any of these alternatives may assist you in integrating other perspectives into communication sciences and disorders.

## Start Looking for a Mentor

Look on a potential university's Web site and, if listed, read about the faculty research pursuits. If there is a professor (or two) whose research interests you, look up some of their peer-reviewed journal articles. Contact the professor via email and explain that you are interested in applying to the Ph.D., Ed.D., or Sc.D. program. Explain what area you are interested in researching and find out more about his or her current projects. Open up a dialog to help determine if this individual might be a good mentor for you.

## Make an Appointment to Speak with the Potential Research Mentor

If your initial contact with a potential mentor goes well, ask for an appointment, either by phone or in person, to speak more extensively about research interests. Inquire about the professor's current research. Find out how many students the professor has mentored in the past and how many he or she is currently mentoring. Ask how long it took the professor to complete his or her Ph.D. The answer may be indicative of how long the Ph.D. program will take you to complete. Ask other questions about the program, the university, and the location so that you have a good understanding of what life would be like if you attend this program.

## Contact Your Undergraduate and/or Master's Program Mentor

Your undergraduate or master's program mentor is a great resource for identifying the right doctoral program for you. Ask for suggestions and advice on finding a doctoral program. Discuss his or her experiences. Remember that this is just one person's opinion, and if you already have a strong personal relationship, your former mentor may be very open and candid, which can help you make informed decisions.

## Thoroughly Research Potential Doctoral Programs

Obtain information from the Web about the programs you are interested in, and do searches of the faculty you are interested in working with. Make personal contact with faculty, as well as current and former doctoral students. The ASHA Web site maintains a list of all ASHA-accredited doctoral programs and general areas of study. A list is also available in Appendix B of this book. Choosing a doctoral program that fits your interests and goals is a very personal decision. Investigate your options thoroughly so you can make decisions that meet your needs.

# Attend the Graduate School Fair at the ASHA Convention

The Graduate School Fair at ASHA's annual convention is a great opportunity for students interested in doctoral programs to meet with faculty. This can give you access to schools across the country that you may not have a chance to visit personally. The NSSLHA and ASHA Web sites provide a listing of programs exhibiting at the Graduate School Fair.

## Visit Potential Doctoral Programs

Make an appointment to visit the department, meet with the professors and possibly clinical supervisors, and speak to any current doctoral students who are available. Feel free to ask them if they will speak to you "off the record" so that you might gain some insider information on how successfully they feel the department functions, or how they feel about their experiences in the program, and so on. (Suggesting an "off the record" discussion implies that what is said by either of you stays between the two of you. Make sure to honor such an agreement.) Contacting and talking to recent graduates can also provide important information.

## When You Visit a Potential Program, Meet with Current Doctoral Students

If you have identified a professor you are interested in working with at a potential program, try to meet with a current doctoral students who are working for him or her. Ask the students how they like working for the professor. What do they like most about the professor? What is sometimes a challenge while working for the professor? What about the research project is interesting and stimulating? What about the project has been challenging? You can also use this meeting to learn more about the environment at the potential program and the resources at the university.

## Ask Questions

The more information you have, the better able you will be to make the right decisions. Contact the program directors or contact persons listed on each Web site of the doctoral programs that interest you. Arrange an interview, either by phone or in person, with that individual and do not hesitate to ask questions, such as:

- Does anyone in the department have any interest in the area of research that I would be interested in?
- Does anyone in related departments have an interest in my area of research?

- How many doctoral students are currently in the program?
- What kind of financial assistance exists for doctoral students? Tuition reimbursement? Research/teaching assistantships? Grants? Scholarships? Conference travel? How stable are the available funding sources? Will there be any obligations attached to funding during my time in the program or after graduation?
- How long does it take most students with my educational background (e.g. bachelor's and/or master's) to graduate?
- May I get a list of current and/or recent alumni to contact about your program?
- Will I be required to study full-time or will I be able to continue working while I study?
- Would I be able to have mentors from outside your department or your academic institution on my committee?
- If I did not complete a master's thesis, will I need to complete an equivalent as a doctoral student?
- Will there be opportunities or obligations to teach undergraduate courses?
- What kind of coursework will I take? Are there required courses? Can I take courses outside the department?
- Does the institution require any culminating projects or comprehensive exams? A culminating project may be a small research study or literature review. Most comprehensive exams are either lengthy tests that take four to eight hours to complete, or they may come in the form of a written exam that requires the student to answer several in-depth questions over several weeks after all coursework and pre-dissertation research projects (if any) have been completed. Either way, the basic goal of this process is to assess the student's knowledge of the field and the specific area of interest obtained up to that point.

## Get Great Letters of Recommendation

Letters of recommendation are critical components to successfully gaining admission and funding to most programs. When applying to doctoral programs, you will need letters of recommendation from persons who can say, based on experience, you will do well in a doctoral program. Contact professors from your undergraduate and/or master's program. If you assisted a professor with research and/or had a research mentor who assisted you with a research project or thesis, ask for a letter of reference. If you have participated in a clinical fellowship, consider asking your CF supervisor. If you have had a direct impact on any of your clients, consider asking them for a letter of recommendation. Choose wisely because these letters typically carry a lot of weight in the admissions process.

## CONCLUSION

By the time you apply to a doctoral program, you probably have gone through the academic application process a number of times and may feel quite comfortable with it. Some of the procedures and requirements are similar to what you may have done before. However, because the level of commitment to a doctoral program is more intense, the information schools are looking for from potential candidates may also be more extensive. As always, locate a program that fits well with your interests and goals. To have the greatest possible chance of gaining admission and funding to your chosen program, determine its specific requirements for admission early and make sure you provide everything needed, as asked for, on or before schedule.

# CHAPTER 21

# Advice for Students in Au.D. Programs

Erica Dmuchoski, 2nd year master's of audiology student, NSSLHA Regional Councilor, Region I, 2001–2003 and Marie Patton, master's student, SLP, University of Wisconsin-Madison and NSSLHA President, 2001–2003

## INTRODUCTION

The Doctorate of Audiology (Au.D.) is a clinical degree that is one of the doctoral degrees that meets the ASHA certification standards, which mandate an earned doctorate for individuals applying for ASHA certification in audiology as of January 1, 2012. Students who enroll in Au.D. programs do not necessarily have a bachelor's degree in Communication Sciences and Disorders; however, students who have a degree in another discipline may have to take some post-bachelor courses on basic speech science and audiology. Most full-time Au.D. programs last four years. The first three years generally consist of coursework and practicum, and the last year of study is a residency.

Every semester will be filled with both classroom hours and clinical hours. Some programs have their own on-campus clinic where experience is gained, while other programs send their students to clinics and hospitals in the area. Typically, programs with on-campus clinics give students opportunities to go to off-campus locations as well. A doctoral project and summer internships are components in Au.D. programs. There are a number of benefits to earning an Au.D.:

- Beginning in 2007, students in audiology will be required to complete 75 post-baccalaureate semester hours of coursework, culminating in a doctoral or some other recognized graduate degree.
- In 2012, ASHA and other professional organizations will only accept audiology members with a doctoral degree. More schooling provides each student with more current knowledge about diagnostics, procedures, and the profession as a whole.
- In contrast with a master's degree (which will not be an option for audiology applicants after December 31, 2006), Au.D. students will have more experience with clients with different pathologies, more practice providing diagnostics and treatment, more exposure to the different work settings, and more opportunities to learn from audiologists who are currently practicing.

This chapter provides a general guideline for what you need to know to succeed in an Au.D. program, and Figure 21-1 provides a checklist to help keep track of your progress.

- [ ] Make sure you are fully knowledgeable about the Au.D. program you are entering.
- [ ] Talk to current students.
- [ ] Ask questions regarding fellowships and/or assistantships.
- [ ] Research financial aid opportunities.
- [ ] Seek out additional resources for audiology students.
- [ ] Take one day at a time.
- [ ] Seek out support.
- [ ] Consider joining different audiology student organizations.
- [ ] Attend the ASHA, NAFDA, and AAA conventions.
- [ ] Once you graduate, maintain your professional affiliations.

**Figure 21-1** Checklist for students in Au.D. programs

## Make Sure You Are Fully Knowledgeable About the Au.D. Program You Are Entering

Be diligent in finding out requirements for graduation and prerequisites for certain courses. Make sure you know what will be expected to successfully graduate from this program and clearly assess whether you can meet the program's standards *before* you enter the program.

## Talk to Current Students

Current students are a fantastic resource for learning about a program, the university, the atmosphere, and the city in which the school is located. If you are attending a program in a new city, make sure that you will be safe on campus. Current students can provide much needed advice on housing and living arrangements. It will be difficult to be a good student if you are worried about your safety. Also ask questions about the cultural offerings and nightlife; after all, your Au.D. will consume at least three years of your life. You are entitled to have some fun and blow off some steam.

## Ask Questions Regarding Fellowships and/or Assistantships

Most Au.D. programs have fellowships, assistantships, and grant programs. Talk with the department chair and representatives in financial aid to find out more about these opportunities and how you can take advantage of them.

Fellowships and assistantships in Au.D. programs are valuable resources for gaining experience while offsetting the costs of your education. Once you are admitted into a program, continue your contact with individuals who are informed about the department's assistantships and fellowships to take advantage of other opportunities as they arise.

## Research Financial Aid Opportunities

Au.D. programs need good students and are often willing to provide financial resources to get them into their program. Exhaust every possible resource in your quest for financial aid and you may even be able to pursue this degree with little money coming out of your own pocket.

## Seek Out Additional Resources for Audiology Students

Go to http://www.audiologystudent.com for resources on issues related to students in audiology. You can participate in student forums on different topics in audiology, search for study guides, and use the glossary. This site also has a peer-mentoring program where, for example, a third-year Au.D. student can serve as a mentor to a senior-year undergraduate student. The site is not affiliated with a university or national organization and there is no fee to use the site. Students can volunteer to edit study guides or for the mentoring program by emailing AuD@audiologystudent.com.

## Take One Day at a Time

The Au.D. program can be demanding. Try to deal with one task at a time; avoid becoming overwhelmed with all that is expected of you. Remember that you are not alone in your situation—your classmates are going through this ordeal with you. Support each other through the process.

## Seek Out Support

Rely on the knowledge and support of second- and third-year students, clinical supervisors, and even fellow classmates. Know that if any problems or issues arise, you can always talk to your program director or clinic director. Do not hesitate to use these people as resources for handling the challenges of the program.

## Consider Joining Different Audiology Student Organizations

Students who are enrolled in Au.D. programs are eligible for membership in NSSLHA, the National Association for Future Doctors of Audiology (NAFDA), and candidate status in the American Academy of Audiology (AAA). Individuals who are members of NSSLHA, NAFDA, and AAA receive great benefits including journals, magazines, newsletters/newspapers, discounts at conventions or conferences (e.g., ASHA and AAA conventions), and scholarship opportunities.

## Attend the ASHA, NAFDA, and AAA Conventions

There are a great many benefits to attending national conventions. This is a great way to meet professionals and learn new techniques in the field. NSSLHA and NAFDA (National Association for Future Doctors of Audiology) members, and candidate members of AAA (American Academy of Audiology) receive a discount to attend conventions. ASHA has also added an Audiology Convention to their programming. For more information on the ASHA convention see Chapter 30.

## Once You Graduate, Maintain Your Professional Affiliations

Individuals with an Au.D. can become members of ASHA and AAA (although additional requirements apply). Check the membership applications for details. Many audiology professionals belong to AAA and/or ASHA because of the benefits, particularly their advocacy power. According to current ASHA membership data, there were 11,566 certified audiology members and 1,250 certified nonmembers in 2003. About 90% of ASHA members are speech-language pathologists/speech scientists and 10% are audiologists/hearing scientists. AAA has 9,000 members (who are audiologists). When these organizations go to Capitol Hill to lobby for legislation that will affect you as an audiologist and/or your clients, they have power in numbers that can make any congressperson more likely to listen. Both organizations are governed by an Executive Board, which is elected by their membership.

## CONCLUSION

One of the most significant changes to the field of audiology is that as of January 1, 2012, individuals applying for ASHA certification in audiology are mandated to hold a doctoral degree in audiology. If you choose to pursue a doctoral degree in audiology, you are likely to hear a great deal about this new certification requirement. If you have questions about the degree requirement or what this means for individuals who are currently practicing professionally with a master's degree, visit the ASHA Web site to learn more. This chapter provides a basic outline of the Doctorate of Audiology. Contact the department chairperson or program director of the programs you are interested in for more detailed information about specific program requirements.

# CHAPTER 22

# Advice for Audiology Students in Sc.D. or Ph.D. Programs

Jeremy Federman, NSSLHA Regional Councilor, Region III, 2003–2005, Caryn Neuvrith, NSSLHA President 2003–2004, Larissa Fedak, NSSLHA Regional Councilor, Region II, 2002–2004, and Marie Patton, master's student, SLP, University of Wisconsin-Madison and NSSLHA President, 2001–2003.

## INTRODUCTION

If you are interested in a research oriented doctorate, the Doctorate of Philosophy (Ph.D.) and Doctorate of Science (Sc.D.) are options. Some Ph.D. programs in audiology offer clinical tracts, but it is best to contact the programs that interest you for more information. Sc.D. programs can be research and/or clinically oriented. Please note that although several Ph.D. programs exist in hearing sciences, only two Sc.D. programs exist and are at Seton Hall University and Boston University. This chapter provides some advice for students in Ph.D. and Sc.D. programs, and Figure 22-1 can be used as a checklist to track your progress.

☐ Consider choosing a research doctoral tract.

☐ Find out if comprehensive exams are required.

☐ Investigate what coursework and research projects are required.

☐ Decide whether to follow the clinical or research doctoral tract.

☐ Investigate the clinical residency requirement.

☐ Prepare for completing a dissertation.

☐ Seek out additional resources for audiology students.

☐ Attend the ASHA and AAA conventions.

☐ Professionally share your research.

☐ Consider applying for student membership in an international organization.

**Figure 22-1** Checklist for audiology students in Sc.D. or Ph.D. programs

## Consider Choosing a Research Doctoral Tract

For individuals enrolled in a Sc.D. program, there is the possibility of pursuing a research doctoral tract, which is a full-time program that includes the same academic coursework, clinical practica, and clinical residency. This tract offers extensive research experiences. These students are required to complete a doctoral dissertation.

## Find Out If Comprehensive Exams Are Required

For Sc.D. and Ph.D. programs, comprehensive exams may have to be taken. Ask your advisor if and when you will be required to take these exams.

## Investigate What Coursework and Research Projects Are Required

The first three years of an Sc.D. program and many Ph.D. programs include courses in basic hearing sciences, such as anatomy and physiology, speech and hearing science, psychoacoustics, and clinical coursework in basic audiometry, hearing aids, auditory evoked potentials, electronystagmography, otoacoustic emissions, and medical audiology. You will be required to take interdisciplinary courses related to scientific and professional writing, statistics, research methods, biomedical ethics, and issues in heath care. Talk with your advisor about the specific coursework of your program. You will also complete a research project or thesis during the first few years. Ask your advisor when you will begin the research project or thesis and what the requirements are for this project. You might want to organize your coursework so that you are taking classes that pertain to your research project first.

## Decide Whether to Follow the Clinical or Research Doctoral Tract

If you are enrolled in a Sc.D. program, decide if you want to take the clinical tract or the research doctoral tract. The research doctoral tract will take at least an extra year. However, if you enjoy research and want to work professionally as a researcher, this tract may be the best choice for you.

## Investigate the Clinical Residency Requirement

The fourth year of a Sc.D. program typically consists of a nine-month clinical residency. If funding is available, the residents are paid a small salary or stipend.

## Prepare for Completing a Dissertation

The fourth and possibly fifth years of a Ph.D. program or research doctoral tract Sc.D. program consists of a dissertation, which is a lengthy research project on a topic that interests you. Work with your program director to determine the specific requirements for your dissertation and be sure to meet those requirements if you want to graduate on time. You will need to defend your dissertation to a dissertation committee as a requirement for obtaining your doctorate.

## Seek Out Additional Resources for Audiology Students

Go to http://www.audiologystudent.com for information and resources on issues related to students in audiology. You can participate in student forums about different topics in audiology, search for study guides, and use the glossary. The site is not affiliated with a university or national organization and there is no fee to use the site. This Web site has a peer-mentoring program where, for instance, a third-year Au.D. student can mentor a senior-year undergraduate student. This is an excellent source of support for undergraduates and a great opportunity for doctoral students to develop their professional skills. Students can volunteer to edit study guides and mentor students by emailing AuD@audiologystudent.com.

## Attend the ASHA and American Academy of Audiology (AAA) Conventions

The many benefits of attending professional conventions are discussed in earlier chapters and in Chapter 30. Conventions are an excellent place to network, learn about issues important to the profession, and to hear current research. If you are a NSSLHA member, you will get the reduced rate at the ASHA Convention. If you already have your CCCs, you still qualify for the reduced rate for graduate students who attend the convention. If you are a candidate member of the American Academy of Audiology, convention registration rates are substantially lower than those for regular members and nonmembers. Additionally, you can apply to be a student volunteer at convention. If selected, your registration is free for providing five to ten hours of work in support of the three-day convention.

## Professionally Share Your Research

You are putting a great deal of work into research as a doctoral student, and you should consider sharing it with your colleagues. Present your work at a poster session at state or national conventions. Submit your written research to a professional journal for publication.

## Consider Applying for Student Membership in an International Organization

There are a number of international, professional organizations that encourage a community to support and disseminate research and that consider important issues in the field of audiology. Membership dues for students are usually less than for regular members, so joining as a student is wise. Some organizations to consider include:

- *Acoustical Society of America (ASA).* This organization is comprised of hearing scientists and some speech scientists, who are interested in speech acoustics. Visit their Web site at http://asa.aip.org for more detailed information about membership fees and activities for students.

- *Association for Research in Otolaryngology (ARO).* This organization is comprised primarily of hearing scientists. Visit the ARO Web site at http://www.aro.org for more detailed information about membership fees and activities for students.

- *American Auditory Society (AAS).* This organization is comprised primarily of hearing professionals. Membership is free if you are a graduate student in audiology or speech and hearing science. Students also receive a free subscription to the journal, *Ear and Hearing*. Visit the AAS Web site at http://www.amauditorysoc.org for more detailed information about the association.

## CONCLUSION

The Ph.D. and Sc.D. degrees are excellent choices for individuals interested in research, and this chapter highlights some of the research oriented aspects of these degrees. As with all degree programs, it is important to know what you want to get out of your doctoral degree so that you can choose a program that most closely fits your personal and professional goals. Once you are accepted into a Ph.D. or Sc.D. program, work closely with your advisor or the chairperson of the department to outline the course of study and requirements for obtaining your degree so that you can graduate on time and begin your professional career.

# Advice for Students in Speech-Language Science Ph.D. Programs

Larissa Fedak, NSSLHA Regional Councilor, Region II, 2002–2004, Sandra Savinelli, SLPD, CCC-SLP, and Marie Patton, master's student, SLP, University of Wisconsin-Madison and NSSLHA President, 2001–2003

## INTRODUCTION

The two types of Ph.D. programs in Speech and Language Science (SLS) are clinically and research oriented. Students can sometimes be accepted into an SLS program with a bachelor's degree if they do not have an interest in gaining clinical experience and want to learn about and conduct research. However, most students in SLS Ph.D. programs have a master's degree in speech-language pathology. A student can apply to a clinical Ph.D. program or to a traditional research Ph.D. program, which does not typically offer clinical experience. There is an alternative research focused degree program called the Doctorate of Speech-Language Pathology (SLPD), which is discussed briefly at the end of this chapter.

This chapter provides a general guideline for what a doctoral program entails. Be sure to check with your potential or current program to see what is required. Generally, most doctoral degrees take four to five years to complete. In most programs, you are a doctoral student until you complete all of the requirements except for your dissertation. After you complete all of the requirements you are considered a doctoral candidate ABD (all but dissertation). Figure 23-1 is a checklist of information covered in this chapter that can be used to keep track of your progress.

## Find Out If Qualifying Exams Are Required

After you are accepted as a doctoral student, you may be required to take the program's qualifying exams in your first year of study. This assures the program that you have the base knowledge to start a doctoral degree. In addition, you

☐ Find out if qualifying exams are required.

☐ Immerse yourself in coursework.

☐ Expect to read (a lot) daily.

☐ Expect to spend hours conducting laboratory research.

☐ Choose a "core" topic.

☐ Learn how to apply for grants.

☐ Form academic/advisory and dissertation committees.

☐ Choose a pre-dissertation topic (if applicable).

☐ At the end of your coursework, take qualifying/comprehensive examinations (if applicable).

☐ Determine whether you are required to complete a research project.

☐ Find out if a master's thesis is required.

☐ Determine if you are using human or animal subjects in your research.

☐ Develop a strong relationship with your advisor.

☐ Determine whether you are required to teach undergraduate courses.

☐ Determine whether you are required to assist a professor in research.

☐ Form relationships with other professors in the department.

☐ Find out if your school has a Preparing Future Faculty (PFF) program.

☐ Complete and defend a dissertation.

☐ Submit your manuscript for publication.

☐ Present your research at a convention.

☐ Join organizations related to your areas of research.

**Figure 23-1** Checklist for students in Speech-Language Science Ph.D. programs

may have to research and write papers on several topics. Sometimes, you will have to speak to a committee about specific topics; these oral exams may take several hours. However, every program is different. Be sure to contact the program director or your advisor to find out what is required.

# Immerse Yourself in Coursework

Now at the highest level of your education, prepare to be immersed in coursework. You will read research journals and texts that will help narrow your focus on a topic or question to investigate in your dissertation. Your advising professor, mentor, and/or advisory committee will assist you in deciding what you will independently study.

# Expect to Read (A Lot) Daily

At this academic level, you will work independently. Be sure to improve your reading skills and maintain your time management skills so that you can stay on top of the independent work you are doing as well as your coursework.

# Expect to Spend Hours Conducting Laboratory Research

The research component of your program will be quite extensive, especially if you are assisting a professor engaged with research in addition to your research project. Hopefully, this is something you are looking forward to, but you should expect to spend a great deal of time working in a lab or setting where research is being conducted.

# Choose a "Core" Topic

As you begin your doctoral study, decide on a core topic area. This will help you with your dissertation. For instance, you could choose Statistics, Interdisciplinary Rehabilitation, or a number of other topics. By taking courses specific to your core, you will be building your knowledge base for your dissertation. Whatever your core area, be sure to take a few statistics courses because they will be useful for critically reviewing journal articles and analyzing your research results.

# Learn How to Apply for Grants

As a research professional, you will need to know how to obtain funding to support your work, and you will likely learn to apply for grants during your doctoral program. Some of the National Institutes of Health (NIH) have funding mechanisms for pre-doctoral experiences. For example, F31 is a National Research Service Award that provides funding during your dissertation. Search the NIH Web site at http://www.nih.gov for Research Training, or speak with the Training and Career Development staff at NIH for details. The U.S. Department of Education (http://www.ed.gov) offers student-initiated research grants. Also check with your university to see if they offer funding for doctoral students.

## Form Academic/Advisory and Dissertation Committees

The academic or advisory committee may help you plan your coursework, research, and other components of your Ph.D. program. The dissertation committee will guide your final research project of your dissertation. A dissertation committee is similar to a thesis committee, and consists of professors from your university who are highly knowledgeable in your area of interest; however it may have more members than a thesis committee. The committee may be cross-disciplinary. For instance, you may choose to have three CSD professors, one psychologist, and one statistics professor. You will choose your dissertation committee based on their expertise and should carefully choose people who can best help you achieve your goals. One of the committee members will serve as the chairperson, and you may work more closely with this individual.

Overall, an advisory or dissertation committee decides what you need to do to graduate with your doctorate. They guide you in deciding what courses to take and monitor your progress on your research. Work closely with your dissertation committee. They are there to assist you through the process of writing your dissertation and will help you graduate in a timely manner. Their goal is to help you become a competent and successful professional who can, in return, add value to the field.

## Choose a Pre-Dissertation Topic (If Applicable)

A dissertation is a major project and can take several years to complete. A pre-dissertation may be like a "pilot" for your dissertation. The pre-dissertation will help you decide if you want to dedicate the next few years of your life to your chosen topic. Equally important, it will help you decide if your research idea is feasible. Talk with your advisor to determine whether this is required or recommended for your program.

## At the End of Your Coursework, Take Qualifying/Comprehensive Examinations (If Applicable)

Your advisory and/or dissertation committee will decide if you are ready and capable to complete a dissertation. If you pass the qualifying/comprehensive examinations, most programs will classify you as a doctoral candidate.

# Determine Whether You Are Required to Complete a Research Project

If you did not complete a master's thesis, you may be required to complete a project that ensures you have the skills needed to complete a dissertation. This project is usually developed with your primary advisor, but each university is different. At some programs, you may complete another research project even if you did one as a master's student. Talk with your advisor to determine what the requirements are for your program.

## Find Out If a Master's Thesis Is Required

Some programs allow students to earn their bachelor's degree and move right into a doctoral program. In these cases, a student may be required to complete a master's level thesis before they can begin their doctoral coursework. Work with your advisor to determine whether this is needed, what is required, and the process for fulfilling the requirement.

## Determine If You Are Using Human or Animal Subjects in Your Research

If you decide to use human or animal subjects in your research, you are likely to need approval from your Institutional Review Board (IRB). This approval is required to ensure the safety of participants in studies, and it is important to adhere to their guidelines. Secure these approvals early so that it will not delay your research.

## Develop a Strong Relationship with Your Advisor

You will need to work closely with your primary advisor throughout the research and dissertation writing/defense process. He or she is your lifeline to help guide you through the doctoral process and gain a solid footing for later professional work.

## Determine Whether You Are Required to Teach Undergraduate Courses

Depending on the nature of your financial aid, scholarships, or assistantships, you may be asked to teach undergraduate courses. If you intend to work in a university setting, it is extremely important that you get teaching experiences as a doctoral student. This is an excellent opportunity for on-the-job training. While you may not have prior teaching experience, you can talk with your advisor, other graduate instructors, and other professors to find ways to develop your teaching skills. When you go to interview for faculty positions, you will be asked questions about your teaching experiences. Be certain to save any student evaluations, especially if they are good ones!

## Determine Whether You Are Required to Assist a Professor in Research

Depending on the nature of your financial aid, scholarships, or graduate assistantship, you may be asked to assist a professor in research. While any research experience is valuable, it is best if you can assist with research directly related to your interests or your dissertation. Talk with your advisor to determine if this is a possibility.

## Form Relationships with Other Professors in the Department

While you may work closely with individual professors on your thesis committee or in your assistantship duties, be sure to develop relationships with other professors as well. They may have contacts in major areas that interest you or have an area of interest that might overlap with your own. Strong relationships with your professors can open doors when you are in the job market.

## Find Out If Your School Has a Preparing Future Faculty (PFF) Program

Many schools have programs, such as a Preparing Future Faculty (PFF) program, or something similar, for students who would like to teach at a university. PFF programs prepare graduate students for teaching in higher education. Most research extensive and intensive universities have a PFF program. Visit http://www.preparing-faculty.org to see if your university has a program. If it does not, see if there is a school nearby. Sometimes, PFF programs allow students to sit in on a PFF course if one is not available at your primary institution.

In addition to providing support and training in classroom instruction, PFF programs explain how to create a teaching portfolio that highlights your teaching philosophy and experiences. Regardless of whether you participate in a PFF program, your teaching portfolio is required when applying for most faculty positions. Have your advising professor review your teaching portfolio before submitting it to job search committees.

## Complete and Defend a Dissertation

At the end of your doctoral program, during which time you have written a dissertation, you will have to defend it to a dissertation committee. The defending of one's dissertation may take several hours and can be a stressful experience, but it can also be very rewarding. If you have been working closely with your dissertation committee, you will be able to predict some of the questions that may be asked about your dissertation. Do not be discouraged if the committee requires some additional work to finalize or polish the dissertation. Hopefully, you will have worked closely enough with your dissertation committee that there will not be any unforeseen delays in passing your work.

## Submit Your Manuscript for Publication

After your dissertation committee has accepted your dissertation, put it into manuscript form and apply for publication in journals. NSSLHA's scholarly journal, CICSD, accepts student's papers. Visit the publication page of the NSSLHA Web site for more information on submitting manuscripts to CICSD. There are a number of other academic journals that may be interested in publishing your work. Talk with your dissertation committee if you are unsure where to start.

## Present Your Research at a Convention

Consider presenting your research at a state convention or the ASHA Convention. Many states allow students and professionals to do a poster session. Contact your state association to find out when the deadline is for submission and what is required. Applications for poster sessions for the ASHA Convention are due in the spring. Visit the ASHA Web site for more details.

## Join Organizations Related to Your Areas of Research

There are a number of organizations devoted to specific topics in SLS that offer support, discussion, and information. Some of these organizations include:

- *Academy of Aphasia.* Primarily has linguists. The Academy of Aphasia holds conventions. Contact the Academy of Aphasia at http://www.academyofaphasia.com for membership details.
- *Linguistic Society of America (LSA).* Primarily has linguists. Contact the LSA at http://www.lsadc.org for more information about membership for students.

## CONCLUSION

This chapter provides a general overview of the process for obtaining a Ph.D. in a Speech-Language Science program. At the beginning of the chapter, an alternative degree is mentioned for students with a master's degree in speech-language pathology who want to improve their clinical skills and expand their experience with research. These students may want to consider a Doctorate of Speech-Language Pathology (SLPD). Currently, the only institution that offers the SLPD is Nova Southeastern University in Florida. The degree is offered via distance learning. Before pursuing this degree, check with the state licensure board where you plan to work to determine the requirements to practice with the SLPD (e.g., for pay scale increases after you complete the program and practice). Figure 23-2 offers some additional advice for students pursuing the SLPD.

- **You will attend a one-time comprehensive orientation** to the program on-campus at Nova Southeastern University.

- **Expect to take at least three years to complete the program.** The maximum amount of time allowed to complete the degree is seven years. During the third year, you will complete an Applied Dissertation (AD).

- **Students are not required to complete clinical hours** if they have a master's degree in speech-language pathology.

- **You will complete courses related to research.** Although the program is not completely geared toward research like Ph.D. programs, research is an important component of the SLPD program.

- **Coursework will focus on expanding your professional knowledge.** For example, you will take courses related to genetics, pharmacology, and advanced voice and swallowing.

- **You will participate in research during the AD process.** For example, some students complete a project and present their findings. Other students complete a literature review.

- **Funding is not readily available from the program.** Students usually seek student loans or grants.

**Figure 23-2** Advice for students in Doctorate of Speech-Language Pathology programs

# CHAPTER 24

## Information about Post Doctorates

### INTRODUCTION

A post doctorate (also referred to as a "post doc") is a unique opportunity for a recent Ph.D. graduate to focus on a specific area of research and strengthen research skills. Post doctorates generally span a period of one or two years and are typically funded by grant money from a faculty member, who serves as the recent Ph.D. graduate's mentor. Participating in post doc research affords the recent Ph.D. graduate opportunities to spend exclusive time on research without teaching, supervising, or committee responsibilities that faculty members typically have.

### PURSUING A POST DOCTORATE

Following are some reasons to pursue a post doc experience:

- To gain more research experience before applying for a tenure faculty position
- To increase the number of articles accepted by peer review publications
- To expand skills and techniques in the research area
- To learn how to effectively organize and manage a lab
- To gain knowledge/experience in a different research area
- To increase funding opportunities with governmental agencies, such as the National Institute of Health (NIH)

### FINDING A POST DOCTORATE POSITION

What is great about a post doc is that the researcher can sometimes create the position under the supervision of a faculty researcher or a clinic. Following is some advice on how to find a post doc position:

- Check university Web sites for listings of post doc positions in the CSD department.
- Consider earning a post doc in a related field, such as psychology or cognitive neuroscience.

- Search the Web sites of organizations, such as the ASHA or NIH.
- Network when going to conventions and conferences. Look for people in your area of interest who have completed a post doctorate or are in charge of a program with a post doctorate position available.
- Ask your advisor from your Ph.D. program for assistance in searching for a post doc position.

## CONCLUSION

If you are on track to receive your doctorate and are interested in research, one of the most valuable experiences you can have is working as a post doctorate. While focusing exclusively on research, you can develop the foundation for presentations and publications and can hone your research skills. Once you take a position as a professor at a college or university, your attention will almost always be divided between teaching and advising responsibilities, committee work and department responsibilities, and research. For many, the post doctorate is a welcome opportunity to devote one's time and attention solely to research.

# CHAPTER 25

# Selected Specialty Interests in Audiology and Hearing Sciences

## INTRODUCTION

Although there are many specialty interests in audiology and hearing sciences, this chapter highlights only some of them. As you will notice, some professionals have more than one area of specialty. This means that, as a student, you will have the opportunity to explore more than one specialty area, if you choose to specialize at all. (Some clinicians choose to be generalists and work with a large spectrum of clients and pathologies.) The following interviews provide a glimpse into audiology and hearing science specialties, including balance and dizziness; cochlear implants; geriatric audiological rehabilitation; health care disparities and cultural competence; amplification, assistive listening devices, and audiological rehabilitation; noise and rehabilitation; and pediatric audiology. The different perspectives and experiences portrayed in this chapter can be useful as you reflect on which areas interest you and are good starting points for investigating specialty areas further.

## BALANCE AND DIZZINESS

An interview with Neil T. Shepherd, Ph.D., CCC-A by Marie Patton, master's student, SLP, University of Wisconsin-Madison and NSSLHA President, 2001–2003. Dr. Shepherd is the ASHA Vice President for Quality Services in Audiology and a professor in the Department of Otorhinolaryngology School of Medicine at the University Pennsylvania.

**Q.** *What made you want to study balance and dizziness?*

**A.** I was trained in biomedical engineering, but my wife was a teacher of the deaf. I wanted to get my Ph.D. in electrophysiology. My background was in control systems.

**Q.** *What are some of the challenges of working within balance dizziness?*

**A.** You have to have an understanding of both perception and motor output control systems. There is a large amount of information to synthesize, typically greater than when dealing with auditory disorders.

With patients, you can get a lot of negative feedback, because patients feel isolated and sedentary. That is compounded with risks for falls. Overall, you have to do counseling because there is a lot of psychological overlay. However, with the appropriate management, you can make significant changes in clients who have had symptoms for months or years.

**Q. How did you become more knowledgeable in your specialty area?**

**A.** I did a lot of outside reading on my own, and I decided that it was an area that I wanted to pursue. At the time, there were zero programs with clinical training in audiology in balance and dizziness. So, for about ten to fifteen years (and still), I did self-studies with individuals from other disciplines. I traveled to meet with people who knew how to do certain things; I learned from them, and they learned from me.

**Q. What populations (e.g., age ranges) do clinicians usually work with within balance and dizziness?**

**A.** You can work with patients from infants up to one hundred year olds.

**Q. What settings might clinicians work in if they specialize in balance and dizziness?**

**A.** Private physician offices to academia, where you may have no contact with patients, doing only research. There's a variety of settings.

**Q. Are there any organizations that provide membership? Do they have any conferences?**

**A.** The Bárány Society (http://www.baranysociety.com/) meets every even year in different locations, usually outside of the U.S. To become a member, two members must nominate you, and there is a review of your vita.

The International Society of Posture and Gait Research has a meeting every odd year. Their Web site is http://www.ispgr.org/.

The meetings for both societies are four intensive days. They are expensive because it's such a small group. However, the expenses pay for most everything.

**Q. What types of skills are needed to work in this specialty area that are not necessary for other areas?**

**A.** A firm knowledge of how the motor system interacts with the input systems of vestibular, proprioception/somatosensory, and vision.

**Q. What are some good resources for students to read who are just getting started in learning about balance and dizziness?**

**A.** ASHA's Knowledge and Skills document in Balance and Dizziness

*The Journal of Vestibular Research*

*The Journal of Otology & Neurotology*
*The Journal of Neurology*
Audiology journals
Multiple books on the subject published since 1996

**Q. *What are the best reasons to work within this specialty area?***

**A.** Balance and dizziness is a very diverse area with a motor aspect. Every medical specialty can potentially see those with disorders of balance and equilibrium. Plus, there's a lot of room for new research.

# COCHLEAR IMPLANTS
•••••••••••••••••••••••••••••••

An interview with Paul J. Abbas, Ph.D., by Marie Patton, master's student, SLP, University of Wisconsin-Madison and NSSLHA President, 2001–2003. Dr. Abbas is a joint professor at the University of Iowa in the departments of Speech Pathology and Audiology and Department of Otolaryngology.

**Q. *What made you want to study electrical stimulation of the ear and cochlear implants?***

**A.** I have a background in engineering and wanted to do something that was more biologically oriented. I took a course in Sound, Speech, and Hearing as an undergraduate and became interested in the auditory system, since it was an area where engineering principles could be applied. After completing graduate school, I was interested in teaching. A faculty position was open in a speech pathology and audiology department to teach and do research in auditory physiology and related topics. After several years doing basic research, primarily with animals, I became interested in cochlear implants. My research now focuses on both basic research on electrical stimulation of the ear and more clinical oriented research with human cochlear implant users.

**Q. *What are some of the challenges of working within these areas?***

**A.** Keeping up with the changes in technology.

**Q. *How did you become more knowledgeable in these areas?***

**A.** Both in graduate school and through meetings, and experience over the years as a faculty member.

**Q. *Are there any specific settings that clinicians work within?***

**A.** Primarily large medical centers.

**Q. *What types of skills are needed to work within cochlear implants?***

**A.** The area of cochlear implants, in general, has many individuals from different disciplines. My particular focus is in electrophysiological measures, where more technical skills are particularly useful.

**Q. *Are there any organizations that provide membership specifically related to cochlear implants?***

**A.** Both the Acoustical Society of America and Association for Research in Otolaryngology have excellent journals and student membership rates.

**Q. *What are some good resources for this area?***

**A.** *The Journal of Acoustical Society of America*
*Hearing Research*
*The Journal of Association for Research in Otolaryngology*
*Ear and Hearing*
*Audiology and Neurotology*

**Q. *What are the best reasons to work with individuals who have cochlear implants?***

**A.** It's a new and changing area in which individuals can be dramatically impacted.

# GERIATRIC AUDIOLOGIC REHABILITATION

Interview with Patricia B. Kricos, Ph.D., CCC-A by Marie Patton, master's student, SLP, University of Wisconsin-Madison and NSSLHA President, 2001–2003. Dr. Kricos is the Director of the Center for Gerontological Studies and Professor in the Department of Communication Sciences and Disorders at the University of Florida.

**Q. *What made you want to work within geriatric audiologic rehabilitation?***

**A.** There were several things that sparked my interest in audiology, particularly geriatric audiology. When I was a young child, I was fortunate to have a grandmother who would read to me every day. One of our favorite books was the story of Helen Keller. The inspiration I received from the book must have coalesced with my deep love and appreciation of my grandmother to ultimately guide me to audiology and gerontology.

**Q. *What are some of the challenges of working within this area?***

**A.** There are a number of challenges of working with elders who are hearing impaired. One is that many of them do not want to wear hearing aids and/or do not realize that they have hearing difficulties. Approximately 80% of elders who potentially might benefit from hearing aids do not use them. In the coming years, it will be of critical importance for audiologists to educate society, as well as individual elders, regarding the effects of hearing loss and rehabilitative options that may be available to assist them.

Another challenge will be the special needs of elders, who often have other chronic conditions besides hearing loss, such as arthritis and visual impairments. The most rapidly growing segment of the American population is the group of elders who are 85 years and older. This group may have special needs that we will need to carefully consider to offer the most useful and relevant intervention to help them lead full lives.

**Q.** *How did you become more knowledgeable in geriatric audiologic rehabilitation?*

**A.** First and foremost was my graduate education at the Ohio State University, where I received my Master's degree and Ph.D. degree in Speech and Hearing Sciences. Early in my graduate work, I was part of a team of speech and hearing researchers who traveled to what was then known as Yugoslavia to learn about a method of audiologic rehabilitation known as the Verbotonal Method. This gave me excellent preparation for working with children who are hearing impaired. My knowledge in the area of geriatric audiology came from a combination of coursework, continuing education, and clinical experiences. Although knowledgeable in my specialty area, I continue to learn more and more about working with elders who are hearing impaired, and I suppose I will continue to learn, long after retirement.

**Q.** *Are there any specific settings that clinicians work within geriatric audiologic rehabilitation?*

**A.** In my specialty area of audiologic rehabilitation of older adults with hearing loss, the primary settings seem to be medical centers, private practices, and Veterans Administration audiology clinics.

**Q.** *What types of skills are needed to work in this specialty area that are not necessary for other specialty areas?*

**A.** Knowledge of the unique communication needs and characteristics of older adults is essential. For example, patient education for this population is so important, so any materials that are prepared need to be useable by this population. The font should be large enough for them to read, mnemonic devices should be provided to help elders and their caregivers remember instructions regarding hearing aids, and consideration of their special needs should be given.

**Q.** *Are there any organizations that provide membership specifically for geriatric audiologic rehabilitation?*

**A.** The Academy of Rehabilitative Audiology (ARA) at http://audrehab.org/ is devoted to the audiologic management across the age spectrum of individuals who are hearing impaired. The primary purpose of the Academy is to promote excellence in hearing care through the provision of comprehensive rehabilitative and habilitative services.

Students who are enrolled at least half time in a program leading to a degree in audiology, speech-language pathology, or education of persons who are hearing impaired can be members. The student members receive the *ARA Newsletter* and the *Journal of the Academy of Rehabilitative Audiology*. One of the best things about being a member of the ARA is the Annual Summer Institute, in which leaders in the field, practitioners devoted to audiologic rehabilitation, and university students can interact and discuss the latest cutting edge research and developments in this specialty.

**Q. *What are some good resources for the specialty area? Are there any journals specific to the specialty area?***

**A.** Some journals that are excellent resources for audiologists who work with elders are the *Journal of the Academy of Rehabilitative Audiology, Journal of Gerontology, The Gerontologist, Generations,* and *International Journal of Audiology.* The more audiologists know about aging, the better prepared they will be to provide effective services to older adults and their families.

**Q. *What are the best reasons to work with this specialty area?***

**A.** The most important reason to work with elders who have hearing loss is that good hearing is so important for achieving quality of life. In a recent survey of senior citizens conducted by the American Association for Retired Persons (2003), 96% of respondents indicated that spending time with family and friends is the most important activity for maintaining quality of life. Research has indicated that hearing loss negatively impacts the communication abilities of older individuals and compromises their quality of life in a number of ways. A large-scale study conducted by the National Council on the Aged (1999) found significantly higher rates of depression, anxiety, frustration, and social withdrawal in seniors with untreated (i.e., no hearing aids) hearing loss. Audiologists, therefore, have an extremely important role to play in helping elders maintain the highest quality of life in their golden years. Every time I conduct Living With Hearing Loss support groups and educational programs for older adults and their family and friends, I have a strong sense of contributing to the overall quality of life, psychological and physical independence, and joy of living of the older adults with whom I work.

# HEALTH CARE DISPARITIES
# AND CULTURAL COMPETENCE
••••••••••••••••••••••••••••••••••••••

Interview with Kenneth E. Wolf, Ph.D., CCC-A by Marie Patton, master's student, SLP, University of Wisconsin-Madison and NSSLHA President, 2001–2003. Dr. Wolf is a member of the ASHA Audiology Legislative Council, Professor, Associate Dean for Educational Affairs, Chair of the Institutional Review Board, and Chief of Audiology at the Charles R. Drew University of Medicine and Sciences in Los Angeles, CA. He is also a former member of the ASHA Multicultural Issues Board.

**Q. *What made you want to study and teach health care disparities and cultural competence?***

**A.** It was really an evolution. The hospital (King/Drew Medical Center) and Charles R. Drew University in South Los Angeles, California, are in one of the poorest, most underserved areas of the country. It's a historically black- and Hispanic-serving institution. More data is coming out that people are not being treated the same way in the health care system. Racial and ethnic minority patients have poorer outcomes than majority patients. In relation to hearing health care, disparities also exist. I want to know how we are going to turn things around in this country. It's bigger than health care, audiology, and speech and language. The health care disparities contribute to the social problems in this country.

**Q. *Why is cultural competence important?***

**A.** Cultural competence goes beyond serving minorities. Everyone has his or her own culture. Everyone has multiple cultures—age, gender, religious background, patient, clinician, etc. You have to make sure that your belief system does not get in the way of providing the best possible service.

**Q. *What are the best reasons to be knowledgeable about health care disparities and to have cultural competence?***

**A.** There's the satisfaction of helping people who have been marginalized and discounted by society. I did some focus groups with people who were minorities and elderly about hearing loss and hearing aids. The individuals were appreciative just to be asked into the focus group and responded, "you were the first ones to ask us what we wanted." It's important to have respect for people. Instead of telling people what to do, talk with them about what they want.

**Q. *What are some of the challenges of working within an environment with individuals who are disadvantaged?***

**A.** While working in a poor and underserved community and hospital, there are never enough resources. You know you can help, but you do not have the hearing aids to help them, or the newest technology to use when you can't quite figure out what's wrong. We are always behind the curve on the new technology because of funding.

**Q. How did you become more knowledgeable in health care disparities and cultural competence?**

**A.** Part of it was clinical experience, asking questions, reading, attending conferences, and talking with colleagues. The more I talked with others at conferences, the more I learned about myself. Learning is a lifelong process.

**Q. What are some good resources for those who want to learn more about health care disparities and cultural competence?**

**A.** The ASHA document, "Knowledge and Skills Needed by Speech-Language Pathologists and Audiologists to Provide Culturally and Linguistically Appropriate Services" is a good resource.

Students can join the ASHA Special Interest Division 14: Communication Disorders and Sciences in Culturally and Linguistically Diverse Populations, and Division 15: Gerontology.

**Q. Is there anything else you would like students interested in this area to know?**

**A.** Go with the flow. Truly, it's the serendipitous nature of one's career. If your path does not go the way you expected it to when you were 20 or 30, look around and see what your options are. Find a way to make a contribution and you will find a reward.

## NOISE AND REHABILITATION

An interview with Laura Ann Wilber, Ph.D., CCC-SLP/A by Marie Patton, master's student, SLP, University of Wisconsin-Madison and NSSLHA President 2001–2003. Dr. Wilber is a member of the ASHA Audiology Legislative Council and Professor Emeritus in Communication Sciences and Disorders at Northwestern University.

**Q. What are your specialty areas? What made you want to work within your specialty areas?**

**A.** In some ways, I have never had a specialty within audiology. I have found the whole field fascinating. However, if I have been locked into specific areas, they have been noise and rehabilitation. Noise, because I was challenged by a non-audiologist friend many years ago (during the era of consideration of supersonic flight) who asked why audiologists were *not* more active in this area. I have not done much in industrial hearing conservation, but into noise in general. Rehabilitation, because I started out in deaf education (before I found audiology) and always had an interest in going beyond the hearing aid fitting.

**Q.** *What are some of the challenges of working within noise and rehabilitation?*

**A.** In noise, most folks don't want to hear about it because they don't notice a problem now; they prefer to think it won't happen to them. This can be frustrating. In rehabilitation, folks don't want to take the time to learn how to communicate better; they want the quick fix. Too many folks seem to still think that putting on a hearing aid should be comparable to putting on eyeglasses. We have not even persuaded all of the folks within our profession to wear hearing aids. So it is not surprising that we haven't convinced the general public.

**Q.** *How did you become more knowledgeable in noise and rehabilitation?*

**A.** Reading, attending short courses and sessions at various conferences.

**Q.** *What populations do clinicians usually work with within noise and rehabilitation?*

**A.** Actually, in both noise and rehabilitation, anyone who has, or might have, a hearing loss is a potential client. In the area of noise, for example, I have testified in court on probable cause of hearing loss, and I have served as a consultant for legal firms concerned about the possibility of noise-induced hearing loss. I have also talked with lay persons (during the first year of Earth Day, for example) about the implications of noise. Anyone with a hearing loss can benefit from aural rehabilitation—that includes the population from birth to adulthood.

**Q.** *Are there any specific settings that clinicians work within noise and rehabilitation?*

**A.** Some clinicians interested in noise, work in industrial areas implementing hearing conservation programs. (That has not been my course of action). Some clinicians do forensic audiology (I have done a little of this, but not a lot). Rehabilitation can be used in all settings.

**Q.** *Are there any special kinds of certification necessary or available for noise and rehabilitation?*

**A.** To work in industrial settings, one needs certification by the Council for Accreditation in Occupational Hearing Conservation (CAOHC) or be supervised by someone with this certification. More information is available on the CAOHC Web site at http://www.caohc.org.

**Q.** *Are there any organizations that provide membership specifically for noise and rehabilitation?*

**A.** In rehabilitation, the primary membership organization is the Academy of Rehabilitative Audiology (ARA). ARA does allow student affiliates. They also have a student award. More information is available on the ARA Web site at http://www.audrehab.org.

In noise, there is probably more information about sound and noise in the Acoustical Society of America, an organization not for audiologists only. It also has student membership. Students can learn more on their Web site at http://asa.aip.org. Another organization to consider in this area is the Council for Accreditation in Occupational Hearing Conservation.

**Q.** *What types of skills are needed to work in noise and rehabilitation that are not necessary for other specialty areas?*

**A.** In noise, one needs a more thorough understanding of sound than is usually taught. In rehab, one probably needs more work in counseling than is usually taught, and much more emphasis on assistive devices than is often given.

**Q.** *What are some good resources for noise and rehabilitation?*

**A.** In noise, there are several journals. The best source is the *Journal of the Acoustical Society of America*. There are several other journals related to noise. In rehab, it is the *Journal of the Academy of Rehabilitative Audiology*. Both of these are peer reviewed. There are others that are not peer reviewed that do have usable information.

**Q.** *What are the best reasons to work within noise and rehabilitation?*

**A.** There is a need to help prevent hearing loss from noise and there is a need to help people who have a hearing loss who cannot be brought back to normal function with hearing aids alone. Both are challenging areas. With possibilities of helping folks with and without hearing loss of all ages, there should never be a lack of professional need in these areas.

## PEDIATRIC AUDIOLOGY

An interview with Richard C. Folsom, Ph.D., CCC-A by Marie Patton, master's student, SLP, University of Wisconsin-Madison and NSSLHA President, 2001–2003. Dr. Folsom is the head of Audiology in the Center on Human Development and Disability. He is an Audiology professor and head of Audiology at the University of Washington-Seattle.

**Q.** *What made you want to work within pediatric audiology?*

**A.** It seems like I've always enjoyed working with children. When I entered the study of Speech and Hearing Disorders, I naturally gravitated toward children. Then, with my first position, I had the opportunity to cover some pediatric clinics. Soon I was covering them all. Since that time, pediatric audiology has been my specialty area.

**Q.** *What are some of the challenges of working within pediatric audiology?*

**A.** Time. It simply takes a great deal more time to do everything. There is no set protocol or procedure that always works. Every evaluation is fluid.

**Q.** *How did you become more knowledgeable in pediatric audiology?*

**A.** First, by attending meetings and communicating with other pediatric audiologists. Following that, I returned to school for my Ph.D. at the foremost pediatric audiology program in the country, the University of Washington. I studied with the top people in this area.

**Q.** *What populations do clinicians usually work with within pediatric audiology?*

**A.** It can range from newborn infants to 18 year olds. But these days, most emphasis is on the early identification of hearing loss, which means a focus on the neonatal period.

**Q.** *Are there any specific settings that clinicians work within?*

**A.** Most likely, pediatric audiology programs are associated with a Pediatric Medical Center or a Pediatric Department within a medical center. Occasionally, pediatric audiology exists as part of a developmental center (although this type of center is usually affiliated with a medical center).

**Q.** *Are there any organizations that provide membership specifically for the specialty pediatric audiology?*

**A.** I don't know of any that specifically provide membership for this specialty area. Most of the larger organizations have subgroups that serve specialty areas and pediatrics is certainly one of them.

**Q.** *What types of skills are needed to work in pediatric audiology that is not necessary for other specialty areas?*

**A.** The type of skills that allow for this fluid approach to assessment; flexibility, the ability and willingness to try a new approach, and the audiologic skills to make changes on the fly.

**Q.** *What are some good resources for pediatric audiology?*

**A.** The main audiology journals have always done a good job in publishing articles in pediatrics. *Ear and Hearing* is a good journal.

**Q.** *What are the best reasons to work in pediatric audiology?*

**A.** It is fun to work with infants and young children. There is a tremendous satisfaction in serving infants and their families and making a difference in their lives.

# AMPLIFICATION, ASSISTIVE LISTENING DEVICES, AND AUDIOLOGICAL REHABILITATION

An interview with Stephanie Davidson, Ph.D., CCC-A by Marie Patton, master's student, SLP, University of Wisconsin-Madison and NSSLHA President, 2001–2003. Dr. Davidson is the ASHA Vice President for Academic Affairs and an Associate Professor in Speech and Hearing Science at The Ohio State University.

**Q. *What made you want to work within amplification, assistive listening devices, and audiological rehabilitation?***

**A.** I entered the field of audiology because I love working with people (especially elderly individuals) and I hoped to be able to help these individuals communicate better. Thus, I think it was natural that I gravitated toward the areas of amplification, assistive listening devices, and audiological rehabilitation. Also, I find it very rewarding that we are able to apply advances in science and technology to devices that can improve communication. For example, as we understand more about how normal and impaired ears function, we are able to apply that knowledge to the development of hearing aids that better serve the needs of our patients.

**Q. *How did you become more knowledgeable in your specialty areas?***

**A.** As is generally the case, I began my education in the classroom/lab and then applied that knowledge in clinical practice. To keep current, I read journals, meet with manufacturers' representatives regarding product developments, and attended conferences. However, I think that one of the best ways to become more knowledgeable is to conduct research. An enormous amount of insight can be gained from critically evaluating past literature and working to extend that knowledge through basic and/or applied research.

**Q. *What populations do clinicians usually work with within these specialty areas?***

**A.** Clinicians can work with all ages—from infants to adults. Clinicians can also work with individuals with a variety of disorders—from congenital hearing loss to presbycusis. But, because the majority of hearing-impaired individuals lost their hearing due to aging (presbycusis) or from a combination of aging and exposure to noise, the largest segment of the population needing hearing aids, assistive devices, and audiological rehabilitation is the elderly.

**Q. *Are there any specific settings that clinicians work within these specialty areas?***

**A.** Clinicians can work in a variety of settings, e.g., private practices, schools, community speech and hearing centers, medical centers, ENT physicians' offices, etc. Clinicians can also choose to work for manufacturers (as in-house consultants or traveling sales representatives).

Clinicians who are interested in research (instead of or in addition to clinical practice) could consider a position in a medical center where research and clinical practice are integrated. Clinicians interested in teaching and research (instead of or in addition to clinical practice) should consider a career as a university professor.

**Q. Are there any organizations that provide membership specifically for these specialty areas?**

**A.** Within ASHA, the Special Interest Division devoted to this area is Division 7: Aural Rehabilitation and its Instrumentation. If students are NSSLHA members, membership in Special Interest Divisions is available at a discounted rate.

There are two other Academies directly related to this area:

- *The Academy of Dispensing Audiologists.* Au.D. students who meet eligibility requirements are able to join for a discounted rate. Students can visit their Web site at http://www.audiologist.org for more information.

- *The Academy of Rehabilitative Audiology.* Student membership is available for a discounted rate and more information is available on their Web site at http://www.audrehab.org.

**Q. What are the best reasons to work within these specialty areas?**

**A.** One reason that the area is rewarding is that it offers a combination of immediate gratification (good patient outcomes in a relatively short period of time after devices are fit) and the chance to develop an ongoing relationship with patients (during on-going counseling or treatment activities).

**Q. What are some of the challenges of working with these specialty areas?**

**A.** One challenge (albeit a good one) is the constant evolution of technology. A clinician must stay on top of what's available to provide the best services to the patients. Another challenge is helping patients realize that we can't bring their hearing back to normal—any device that we fit, must still deliver the signal to an impaired auditory system for processing.

**Q. Are there any special kinds of certification necessary or available for these specialty areas?**

**A.** In most states, a license is required to fit hearing aids and assistive devices. The authority to fit these devices might be included in the general audiology license; but some states may require an additional license or certificate.

**Q. What are some good resources for this specialty area?**

**A.** The Web sites of the product manufacturer's are often good resources in the area. Two "trade" journals also can be valuable resources: *The*

*Hearing Journal* and *The Hearing Review.* Other journals specific to the specialty area are *Trends in Amplification* and *Journal of the Academy of Rehabilitative Audiology.*

## CONCLUSION

The audiologists and hearing scientists interviewed in this chapter offer a glimpse into the different specialty areas in which you may want to work. If a particular specialty area interests you, consider contacting local audiologists and hearing scientists about conducting an interview of your own. Speaking with an experienced professional is a great way to get an inside view of what life is like working in that setting.

# CHAPTER 26

## Selected Specialty Interests in Speech-Language Pathology and Speech-Language Sciences

## INTRODUCTION

This chapter provides interviews with professionals with a variety of perspectives and experiences working in selected specialty interests in speech-language pathology and speech-language sciences. This collection of specialty interests is by no means exhaustive, and you are encouraged to investigate these and other specialty areas further. In this chapter, CSD students interviewed clinicians and researchers to learn why they entered into their specialty interest and why the specialty interest is so important to them. While the reasons one chooses a specialty interest are as varied as the individuals themselves, hopefully the interviews in this chapter will help you begin considering whether there is an area that you want to specialize in, or if you would prefer to be a generalist and work with a variety of pathologies and conditions.

## CLEFT LIP AND PALATE SPECIALTY

An interview with Claudia A. Magers, MS, CCC-SLP by Marie Patton, master's student, SLP, University of Wisconsin-Madison and NSSLHA President, 2002–2003. Ms. Magers is a clinical speech-language pathologist at Children's Mercy Hospital and associate professor. She has been a committed ASHA member since 1979.

**Q. *What populations do clinicians usually work with within the cleft lip and palate specialty?***

**A.** We can work with children and adults who have had a facial cleft including children whose clefts have been repaired, but remain velopharyngeally inadequate. They may continue to display hypernasality and nasal air emissions, and possible compensatory articulation errors. These children and adults need additional assessment and possible treatments. Children with craniofacial disorders and certain syndromes may have more of a tendency to display speech disorders related to these areas.

**Q.** *Are there any specific settings that clinicians work within the cleft lip and palate specialty?*

**A.** A clinical environment, where there is a cleft palate-craniofacial team, will provide the most 'accessible' setting. Ours is associated with Children's Mercy Hospitals & Clinics, Hearing & Speech, Plastic Surgery, and Dental departments. Our team also provides multiple professionals to assist in the team evaluations in audiology, speech-language, plastics, dental, ear/nose/throat, pediatrics, nursing, nutrition, occupational therapy, lactation, social services, genetics, and other professionals, depending on the child's needs.

**Q.** *What made you want to work within your specialty area? What sparked your interest?*

**A.** I was working on a degree in speech and drama originally. I heard a young man who was very difficult to understand read a suicide note that he had written while in high school. He tried, unsuccessfully, to commit suicide, because he was made fun of, due to his speech. I started asking questions to some of my professors about why people have speech problems, and who helps them? I was challenged to do an independent study on "Speech Correction," which I completed during the summer of my junior year of college. The more I studied, the more I came to realize that this young man had suffered from a cleft lip and palate, with residual speech effects. After graduation from college with a speech and drama degree, I started investigating the field of speech-language pathology, and the rest is history!

I didn't originally pursue cleft palate as a specialty; but, I have had the privilege, here at Children's Mercy Hospitals & Clinics, to continue to pursue knowledge and experience with this special population. The more I learned, and the more I worked with these children, the more I had a desire to "be the best" SLP in this area that I could be.

**Q.** *How did you become more knowledgeable about cleft lip and palate?*

**A.** I have read just about every book that was ever printed on cleft palate, I think. I continue to buy books and read them, as there always seems to be more to learn. In addition, I have had the privilege to pursue continuing education by attending the annual meetings for the American Cleft Palate Craniofacial Association (ACPA). There have been wonderful mentors at ACPA throughout the years that have willingly shared their knowledge and experiences. The next best thing is to work with these children directly in both assessment and treatment. Nothing teaches you as well as having to figure out what is wrong, and what is the best way to help fix it! The majority of my treatment caseload for over the last 15 years has been with the cleft palate population.

**Q. *What are some of the challenges of working with the cleft lip and palate specialty area?***

**A.** Not all outcomes are the "best." Sometimes you have to admit to the family that you have done all you can do. Working with children can often be difficult, as they can be very stubborn at times, and some of the assessments I do are "invasive," which increases the challenge with a 'difficult' child. Finding funding for long-term treatment needs is always challenging! And finding time to work everyone in is often challenging. Some families drive several hours to come for the evaluations. When recommending treatment, it is often a challenge to find qualified SLPs who are willing and able to provide quality treatment for this specialty area.

**Q. *What types of specific skills are needed to work in the cleft lip and palate specialty area?***

**A.** A good underlying and workable knowledge of anatomy and physiology of the head & neck; a strong understanding of the effects of clefting upon communication, particularly in regards to velopharyngeal functioning/ dysfunction; excellent rapport with children of all ages, and their families; patience; ability to win the trust and cooperation from even the most difficult child; and a thorough understanding of the principles of speech treatment for cleft palate speech.

**Q. *Are there any special kinds of certification necessary or available for this specialty area? Is there an ASHA Special Interest Division?***

**A.** I think ASHA is considering some specialty certifications, one of which will be in the area of physical disorders and effects on speech. Students with an interest in this area should consider membership in Division 5: Speech Science and Orofacial Disorders.

**Q. *Are there any organizations that provide membership specifically for this specialty area?***

**A.** The American Cleft Palate-Craniofacial Association (ACPA), http://www. cleftpalate-craniofacial.org, accepts membership from students and includes reduced dues and registration fees for the annual scientific convention. Student members pay a reduced annual member fee with no entrance fee requirement. Student membership may be granted to an applicant whose professional interests are consistent with the goals of the Association, who has displayed an interest in the study or treatment of cleft lip/palate or other craniofacial anomalies, and who is a full-time student in good standing in an undergraduate, graduate, or post-graduate training program. Students receive a subscription to the *Cleft Palate-Craniofacial Journal*, and receive the ACPA/Craniofacial-Palate Foundation (CPF) newsletter.

**Q.** *What are some good resources for the cleft lip and palate? Are there any journals specific to this specialty area?*

**A.** The ACPA has a journal, *American Cleft Palate-Craniofacial Association Journal*. More information is available on their Web site.

The best comprehensive book out there right now for a new student to this field is *Cleft Palate Speech, 3rd ed.*, published by Mosby. The authors are S. Peterson-Falzone, M. Hardin-Jones, and M. Karnell, copyright 2001.

Another good resource for understanding the philosophy of treatment is *Therapy Techniques for Cleft Palate Speech & Related Disorders* by Karen J. Golding-Kushner, published by Singular/Thomson Delmar Learning, copyright 2001.

**Q.** *What are the best reasons to work with this specialty area?*

**A.** For me, it is because I can see that I can really make a difference! I love this specialty! And I love the children and families I am able to serve. I can see that it changes lives forever!

# CHILD LANGUAGE, AUGMENTATIVE AND ALTERNATIVE COMMUNICATION (AAC), CHILDREN WITH SEVERE/PROFOUND DISABILITIES NEEDING SIGNIFICANT SUPPORT, AMERICAN SIGN LANGUAGE (ASL), AND DRUG-EXPOSED INFANTS AND TODDLERS

An interview with Jeanne M. Johnson, Ph.D., CCC-SLP by Nichole Castle, master's student in SLP at Eastern Washington University. Dr. Johnson is an ASHA certified speech-language pathologist and an undergraduate coordinator for the Department of Speech and Hearing Sciences at Washington State University.

**Q.** *What populations do clinicians usually work with within your areas of specialty?*

**A.** For AAC and severe disabilities interests, clinicians work with individuals who have congenital and acquired disabilities, who are nonverbal, or minimally verbal, and need augmented means of communicating. For ASL, the population is individuals who are deaf and use ASL. Some have deaf parents, and some have hearing parents. Some individuals learned ASL from birth, whereas others were exposed later in life. For children who were drug-exposed, my research focus has been on children prenatally exposed to cocaine or other drugs, including nicotine, alcohol, heroin, marijuana, amphetamines, and prescription drugs.

**Q. *What made you want to work within your specialty areas? What sparked your interest?***

**A.** I worked in the public schools for nine years before pursuing my Ph.D. During that time in the schools, I focused increasingly on children with severe disabilities and children who were deaf. I wanted to know more about language and communication, so I went back to school at the urging of Barry Prizant, who had put on a workshop at Central Washington University about the then-new "Transactional Model" in the area of AAC. The American Sign Language (ASL) interest comes from my family. My grandparents were deaf and my mother, who is hearing, has been involved in the Deaf community and was Washington State Coordinator for Deaf Services prior to her retirement. The drug-exposure interest came from my focus on parent-child interactions, language development, and the "news of the day," which claimed drug-exposed children were "doomed." When I started that research, there were few data to support or refute such claims.

**Q. *How did you become more knowledgeable about this specialty areas?***

**A.** I left my cushy job as an itinerant SLP and went to Southern Illinois University-Carbondale to work with Barry Prizant, Mike Crary, Dennis Molfese, and then, Ken Ruder. My dissertation was focused on cerebral lateralization for linguistic versus nonlinguistic stimuli in congenitally deaf adults who were ASL users. After I completed my Ph.D., I went to the University of Kansas as a post doctoral fellow to work with Mabel Rice in the Child Language Program. During all of this, I did private consulting with families of children with severe disabilities who needed augmentative communication. As for the drug-exposure interest, I became knowledgeable by doing literature reviews, attending conferences, and consulting with professors here at Washington State University (WSU) who were doing research on drug addiction. I received a grant from the WSU Alcohol and Drug Abuse Program, a research incubator, then another, and then became the Interim Director of the Program while we searched for a permanent director.

**Q. *What are some challenges with this area?***

**A.** The biggest challenge is figuring out how to apply all that I know in an individualized manner to a child and his or her family, such that it leads to meaningful and functional outcomes for everyone. The next biggest challenge is working with teams so that the intra-team dynamics facilitate progress for the child.

**Q. *What types of skills are needed to work in this specialty areas?***

**A.** For AAC, one needs to be aware of the new products on the market and how they might be used with various clients. For the other areas, the basics of child language are applicable.

**Q.** *Are there any special certifications necessary or available for this specialty area?*

**A.** Not at this time, although, there has been discussion of an AAC specialty certificate within ASHA.

**Q.** *Are there any organizations that provide membership for this area?*

**A.** ASHA has Special Interest Divisions for Child Language (Division 1) and AAC (Division 12). NSSLHA members can join a special interest division at a reduced fee.

**Q.** *Are there any journals specific to this area?*

**A.** The resources for child language and children with disabilities are numerous and include all of the ASHA journals, JASH, *Mental Retardation, Child Development, Infant Behavior & Development, Journal of Communication Disorders, Seminars in Speech & Language,* and *Topics in Language Disorders,* to name a few. For AAC, there is the fine journal, *Augmentative & Alternative Communication,* as well as some technology-related journals. For ASL, there are journals such as *Sign Language Studies, American Annals of the Deaf,* newsletters from Gallaudet University, and numerous texts. In the area of drug exposure, I use Medline searches because there are so many journals in which to find articles.

**Q.** *What are the best reasons to work within this specialty area?*

**A.** You get to play with babies and get paid for it! Seriously, there is nothing more complex than children with disabilities and their families. There are endless variations on contributing factors to the underlying etiology. The challenges are stimulating and motivating for me.

## NEUROGENICS

An interview with Candace Vickers, MS, CCC-SLP by Marie Patton, master's student, SLP, University of Wisconsin-Madison and NSSLHA President, 2001–2003. Candace Vickers is an ASHA-certified speech-language pathologist in the Outpatient Neurological Rehabilitation Services at St. Jude Medical Center. She is the founder and group leader of communication recovery groups for persons with aphasia at the center and also a part-time instructor at California State University.

**Q.** *What populations do clinicians usually work with within neurogenics?*

**A.** The specialty area includes working with both children and adults who have neurogenically-based language, cognitive, and/or motor speech disorders. Clients may have visual deficits, hearing impairment, and/or dysphagia as well. In addition, many clients will need augmentative communication devices. Finally, there is a great need for clinicians to provide family education and training in conjunction with direct services for the client.

**Q. *Are there any specific settings that clinicians work in within this specialty area?***

**A.** Settings include hospitals, rehabilitation centers, skilled nursing facilities, homes, community-based clinics, day treatment centers, university training clinics, centers for students with disabilities in community colleges, and school settings.

**Q. *What made you want to work within neurological services? What sparked your interest?***

**A.** I was fascinated by what I learned in my graduate neuropathology course about brain functioning and the ability of a well-trained speech-language pathologist to relate symptoms and behavior to a site of lesion. I found the "detective work" aspect of the job especially challenging, which captured my initial interest. I subsequently fell in love with working with persons with neurogenic communicative disorders, and have focused most of my career on working with adults with aphasia. Throughout my career, I have been most influenced by the Minor Hemisphere Mediation model of treatment. I have found it challenging and fascinating to seek to facilitate right brain involvement in tasks to encourage left hemisphere functioning for those individuals affected by aphasia.

**Q. *How did you become more knowledgeable in your specialty area?***

**A.** While still a graduate student, and after completion of my medical internship, I was fortunate to apply for and be accepted as a speech pathology trainee at the Long Beach Veterans Administration (V.A.) Hospital. I spent 15 months working 20 hours a week as a trainee and had the opportunity to not only observe expert clinicians working with a variety of challenging cases, but also to have my own caseload of adults with both language and motor speech disorders. In addition to this very valuable extra experience, I also had the opportunity to attend brain cuttings in the morgue, as well as neurology rounds where cases were discussed on a weekly basis. I was also fortunate to have the opportunity to conduct my graduate project with three discharged patients with aphasia and receive expert guidance in statistical analysis from a valued colleague. Throughout my years in the field, I have been an avid reader of the literature concerning my interest area and attended conferences whenever possible. Finally, I was fortunate to have pursued additional education in counseling psychology, and this knowledge base has served me well in working with both individuals with communication disorders and their families.

**Q. *What are some of the challenges of working with this specialty area?***

**A.** I believe that clinicians that choose to specialize in treatment of this population should be very motivated to pursue lifelong learning through a variety of means. Reading and attending educational offerings take extra time and commitment, but are well worth it. Clinicians need to have a good overall understanding of anatomy and physiology of the central nervous system and be able to discern brain and behavior relationships. Clinicians will experience the joy of providing assistance, but also the pain of loss in dealing with this very vulnerable population. I believe clinicians need the ability to discern how the "cup is half full" and capitalize on every small bit of potential that exists to help individuals who may be severely physically impaired. An additional challenge—which has lasted nearly a decade—is providing the needed amount and duration of services to clients even though health care reimbursements have been shrinking. Finally, knowledge of counseling and crisis intervention techniques is very helpful.

**Q. *What types of skills are needed to work in these specialty areas that are not necessary for other specialty areas?***

**A.** As mentioned earlier, clinicians need a good working knowledge of the central nervous system. They need an expertise in differential diagnosis so that they can provide information to physicians and team members working with the client. Special diagnostic skills in assessment of dysphagia, including the ability to conduct both bedside and Modified Barium Swallow tests are essential for those working in a medical setting. An additional new skill for those working with dysphagia involves being certified in VitaStim. Finally, I believe a background in counseling is essential, since so many of the persons one sees are in great emotional pain.

**Q. *Are there any special kinds of certification necessary or available for the specialty area? What is necessary for certification?***

**A.** There is currently no mandatory certification needed beyond having one's Certificate of Clinical Competence (CCCs). However, it is possible to become board certified by experts in the field through the Academy of Neurological Communication Disorders and Sciences (ANCDS), http://www.ancds. duq.edu.

**Q.** *Are there any organizations that provide membership specifical-ly for neurogenics? Do you know if they allow student affiliates? Do you know the cost to join or their Web site?*

**A.** ASHA Division 2, the Special Interest Division for Neurophysiology and Neuroscience of Neurogenic Communication Disorders, encourages stu-dents to become affiliates. Students will receive four top quality newslet-ters each year that contain articles written by experts in the field about a wide range of issues concerning assessment and treatment of both chil-dren and adults. Affiliates also receive discounts for short courses at the ASHA Convention. ASHA Division 2 also sponsors a free listserv in which clinicians can discuss cases and provide input to others.

**Q.** *What are some good resources for this specialty area? Are there any journals specific to this specialty area?*

**A.** Membership in Division 2 is essential. Memberships in the Gerontology (Division 15) and Dysphagia (Division 13) Special Interest Divisions are also very helpful. Clinicians should subscribe to both the *American Journal of Speech Language Pathology* and *Journal of Speech Hearing and Language Research*. Access to the *Aphasiology* journal is invaluable. Other helpful journals include the *Journal of Medical Speech Language Pathology, Journal of Communication Disorders*, and the *International Journal of Communication Disorders*.

**Q.** *What are the best reasons to work with this specialty area?*

**A.** The ability to use communication is part of what Roberta Chapey has called the "human essence." For me, I cannot imagine a more fulfilling type of work. To help individuals and their families be able to experience the most fulfilling lives possible by assisting in communication is incred-ibly challenging and rewarding. It is never boring!

# CHILDREN WITH MEDICALLY COMPLEX CONDITIONS

An interview with Lemmietta G. McNeilly, Ph.D., CCC-SLP by Barbara Cardeso, NSSLHA member, Florida International University. Dr. McNeilly is a department chair and Associate Professor at Florida International University. She is an ASHA-certified speech-language pathologist.

**Q.** *What populations do clinicians usually work with within this specialty area?*

**A.** The population that most SLPs work with include children with cleft palates, respiratory diseases, cardiopulmonary diseases, HIV/AIDS, as well as genetic disorders.

**Q.** *Are there any specific settings that clinicians work within this specialty area?*

**A.** Yes, these settings include pediatric specialty hospitals, both acute and rehabilitation.

**Q.** *What made you want to work within your specialty area?*

**A.** Children with medically complex conditions are quite diverse with respect to the types of communication disorders they exhibit. Each case presents a unique set of conditions and questions to be answered by clinicians.

**Q.** *What sparked your interest?*

**A.** I worked with children at a rehabilitation hospital in Washington, DC, and I was fascinated by the complexity of the infants and toddlers that I worked with across the hospital. I was most intrigued by the infants and toddlers that exhibited language and/or swallowing difficulties. The interdisciplinary team approach that we utilized was a successful model.

**Q.** *How did you become more knowledgeable in your specialty area?*

**A.** By attending workshops, reading numerous journal articles, books, and working as a member of interdisciplinary teams in several hospitals. Therefore, I increased my knowledge with both information and experience.

**Q.** *What are some of the challenges of working with this specialty area?*

**A.** There are several challenges including the complexity of the disorders in one child, the need to apply culturally appropriate assessment and intervention strategies, and to educate families about the communication disorders and accessing services in different venues.

**Q.** *What types of skills are needed to work in these specialty areas that are not necessary for other specialty areas?*

**A.** In addition to meeting the ASHA certification requirements, clinicians need to be knowledgeable about the medical conditions and the effects of medications on the child's communication functioning. Clinicians need to be competent in working with families and children from culturally and linguistically diverse backgrounds, and have experience working with infants, toddlers, and children with respiratory problems, tracheostomies, and other medical conditions.

**Q.** *Are there any special kinds of certification necessary or available for this specialty area?*

**A.** Some hospitals require clinicians to have Neurodevelopmental (NDT) certification, but currently ASHA does not have specialty recognition for pediatric neurogenics.

**Q.** *Are there any organizations that provide membership specifically for this specialty area?*

**A.** ASHA has Special Interest Division 1: Language Learning and Education. There is also the Council for Exceptional Children (CEC) and the Division for Early Childhood (DEC). The ASHA Special Interest Divisions accept student affiliate members. More information about Division 1 is available on the Special Interest Division page of the ASHA Web site.

**Q.** *What are some good resources for this specialty area?*

**A.** The ASHA position statements, practice guidelines, and technical reports; PubMed; journals; and books in Medical Speech Language Pathology including:

Golper, L. A. (1997). *Sourcebook for medical speech pathology.* San Diego, CA: Singular Publishing Group, Inc.

Vogel, D., & Carter, J. (1998). *The effects of drugs on communication disorders.* San Diego, CA: Singular Publishing Group.

Miller, R., & Groher, M., (1998). *Medical speech pathology.* Gainesville, FL: Contemporary Program.

Johnson, A., & Jacobson, B. (1998). *Medical speech-language pathology: A practitioner's guide.* New York: Thieme.

McNeilly, L. Documentation requirements for pediatric hospital based programs. *Contemporary issues in communication sciences and disorders: Documentation across service delivery settings.* Rockville, MD: NSSLHA.

**Q.** *Are there any journals specific to this specialty area?*

**A.** Yes there are: the *Journal of Medical Speech-Language Pathology, Pediatrics,* and the *Journal of American Medical Association* (JAMA).

**Q.** *What are the best reasons to work with this specialty area?*

**A.** The children are challenging and rewarding. Working with children and families from culturally and linguistically diverse backgrounds allows clinicians the opportunity to enhance clinical skills and to formulate clinical research questions.

# FLUENCY

An interview with Gordon Blood, Ph.D., CCC-SLP by Kelly Farquharson, NSSLHA Regional Councilor, Region I, 2003–2005. Dr. Blood is a professor in stuttering and Program Director for Communication Science and Disorders at Pennsylvania State University.

**Q.** *What made you want to work within the area of stuttering?*

**A.** After studying on the West Coast of Africa in Ghana my junior year in college, I realized the critical nature of communication, as well as the impact of disordered communication, especially stuttering. While living with a family in Kumasi, Ghana, my host family's youngest son stuttered severely. He was continually mocked and the brunt of numerous pranks. This touched me very deeply and I wanted to find a way to help individuals who stutter. When I returned to the United States, I started investigating the field of stuttering and was fascinated by the conflicting information and theories. I decided when I entered graduate school that not only would I try to answer some of the critical questions, but also develop better ways of treating and assisting people who stutter to improve the quality of their lives through more effective communication.

**Q. *What areas are you researching?***

**A.** Most recently, I am looking at the psychosocial aspects (self-esteem, communicative competence, bullying, etc.) in adolescents who stutter. My previous research has examined auditory dysfunction and its relationship to stuttering.

**Q. *How long have you been involved in research in this area?***

**A.** I decided to pursue a Ph.D. in order to acquire the knowledge and skills necessary to answer questions in the areas of stuttering and voice and to use this information to help individuals with communication disorders. I've had my Ph.D. for 26 years.

**Q. *What would you want students to know about your area of interest? What are some of the challenges?***

**A.** Stuttering is probably one of the most complicated and complex areas of our discipline. Attempting to help people who stutter involves "true" interdisciplinary teams and individuals committed to an understanding of the behavioral, attitudinal, and cognitive processes involved. The three million people who stutter in the United States daily confront unbelievable barriers of stereotyping and prejudice and yet somehow manage to cope effectively and become effective communicators. It never ceases to amaze me whenever a client enters therapy, the level of courage and willingness to confront their own fears/avoidance in their quest for effective and competent communication. After reading about, listening to, and working with children, adolescents, or adults who stutter, how could someone not want to research and study this area?

**Q. *What advice do you have for students considering research in this area?***

**A.** Unfortunately, camps or silos have been set up in the field of stuttering that categorize the disorder by etiology, treatment, etc. My suggestion for students considering research in this area is to remain open to all possibilities. In a few years, technology has taken us from dichotic listening tests to positron emission topography (PET) scans and allowed us a closer examination of hemispheric processing or subtle changes in the brain.

Researchers who ignore the possibility of one etiology over another, refuse one type of treatment over another, or one type of assessment over another really limit their ability to answer the big questions in this area. The need for researchers to appreciate diverse contributions from multiple disciplines will allow the true beneficiaries, people who stutter, to make positive changes in their lives and to allow them greater educational, vocational, and social opportunities.

**Q. *Any other comments/suggestions you would like students to know?***

**A.** The best piece of advice provided to me by a mentor was simply to "follow your passion." If students have a strong desire to improve the quality of people's lives through more effective communication, the research questions will flow and the passion needed to answer them by designing and executing important studies will follow.

# NEUROGENIC SPEECH AND LANGUAGE PATHOLOGIES: APHASIA AND APRAXIA

An interview with Malcolm R. McNeil, Ph.D., CCC-SLP by Kelly Farqhuarson, NSSLHA Regional Councilor, Region I, 2003–2005. Dr. McNeil is a professor and Chair of the Department of Communication Science and Disorders at the University of Pittsburgh. He is also the recipient of the 2003 NSSLHA Honors Award, the highest honor bestowed by the association, for his outstanding work with students in CSD programs.

**Q. *Why did you choose to research neurogenic speech and language pathologies in CSD?***

**A.** I chose communication science and disorders as a vocation because it is socially important, offers a one-on-one therapeutic environment, and it is as challenging as any area of health care. It is the clearest and most comprehensive window into the brain and the mind, and one can never know enough to research or treat the vast array of problems confronting persons with communication disorders.

**Q. *What disorders do you study within neurogenic speech and language pathologies?***

**A.** The disorders that I personally study—not all of those represented by the areas of specialization by any means—are primarily, though not exclusively, aphasia and apraxia of speech.

**Q. *What are some challenges of working in neurogenics?***

**A.** One must know everything about sensorimotor speech production, language, and all of the cognitive mechanisms that support language and speech. Additionally, all of the auditory and visual systems (neurologic and cognitive) are implicated in all of these disorders. Current psycholinguistics and neuropsychology are the foundation for studying and understanding both areas and one must know all that is going on in these areas in order to be on the cutting edge of research.

**Q. *What types of skills are needed to work within neurogenics that are not necessary for work in other specialty areas?***

**A.** One needs a firm grasp on neurology and neuropathology, as well as current models of cognitive psychology and psycholinguistics. The landscape is broad and the tilled grounds are deep and filled with rocks.

**Q. *Are there any special kinds of certification necessary or available for neurogenics?***

**A.** The Academy of Neurologic Communication Sciences and Disorders provides specialty certification for those qualifying in either or both adults and children. There is a rather rigorous procedure for demonstrating competencies.

**Q. *Are there any organizations that provide membership specifically for neurogenics?***

**A.** The Academy of Neurologic Communication Sciences and Disorders, http://www.ancds.duq.edu, provides membership at several levels. There is also the ASHA Division 2: Neurophsyiology and Neurogenic Speech and Language Disorders.

**Q. *What are some good journals for those who want to read more about neurogenics?***

**A.** There are *many* journals specific and relevant to this area of specialization. Some of the most popular and frequently cited are *Aphasiology*, *Brain and Language*, and *Journal of Medical Speech Language Pathology*.

**Q. *What advice do you have for students considering research in this area?***

**A.** My advice is to pick a topic within neurogenic communication science and disorders and read everything you can about it and everything that you can about areas that may impact it. Everything you learn about the topic and the methods of investigating it will generalize to anything else that captures your interest

**Q. *Do you have any other suggestions for students?***

**A.** Pick a topic to study and stick with it until you have figured it out. When you have, you will be able to look back at retirement and with the satisfaction of perseverance, know that you have made a contribution.

# ENVIRONMENTAL AND CULTURAL INFLUENCE ON CHILDREN'S LANGUAGE AND LITERACY DEVELOPMENT

• • • • • • • • • • • • • • • • • • • • • • • • • • • • • • • • • •

An interview with Carol Scheffner Hammer, Ph.D., CCC-SLP by Kelly Farquharson, NSSLHA Regional Councilor, Region I, 2003–2005. Dr. Hammer is a professor of child language at Pennsylvania State University.

**Q. *What are your areas of interest?***

**A.** My research focuses on the environmental and cultural influences on children's language and literacy development, with emphasis on African American and Latino/bilingual populations. I am interested in using the information gained through my research to help clinicians better understand the families they work with and to assist clinicians to tailor their interventions to individual families.

**Q. *Why did you choose these areas?***

**A.** My interest in this area stems from my clinical experiences working with families and children. More specifically, I spent two years working as an SLP in Micronesia, where I needed to adapt my approach to service delivery to a very different population. The goal of my research is to understand how caregivers guide their children's development based on norms and expectations of their communities and cultures, and to use this information to assist clinicians to develop practices that build from families' perspectives about parenting and language development.

**Q. *How long have you been involved in research in this area?***

**A.** My work in this area started during my doctoral program. My dissertation focused on how African American mothers of low socio-economic status (SES) and middle-SES supported their children's language development.

**Q. *How long did you wait between earning your master's degree and returning for doctoral work?***

**A.** Eight years. Prior to returning for my doctorate, I worked clinically in schools, early intervention programs, and private practice.

**Q. *What would you want students to know about your area of interest?***

**A.** This area of research draws on information from a variety of disciplines, such as psychology, sociology, anthropology, and education, which makes it an exciting area to be involved in.

**Q. *What advice do you have for students considering research in this area?***

**A.** If you are interested in pursuing research in this area, or in any area in the field, it is important to identify a mentor who shares common research interests and who has an established line of research in the area. Often, students think of choosing a particular university when applying to Ph.D. programs; however, it is equally important to find a faculty member who can guide one in one's area of interest.

**Q. Do you have any more suggestions for students?**

**A.** I would encourage students to strongly consider entering a Ph.D. program if they have an interest in research. A wonderful benefit of being a Ph.D. is that one continues to develop and acquire knowledge throughout the course of his or her career.

# DYSPHAGIA
●●●●●●●●●●●●●●

An interview with Nancy Swigert, MA, CCC-SLP by Marie Patton, master's student, SLP, University of Wisconsin-Madison and NSSLHA president, 2001–2003. Ms. Swigert is the owner of Swigert & Associates, Inc., an ASHA Fellow, President of the American Speech-Language-Hearing Foundation, and former ASHA President.

**Q. What made you want to work within dysphagia?**

**A.** I like the fact that dysphagia is tied closely to medical diagnoses and there is a lot of diagnostic work. I am intrigued figuring out the nature and cause of a problem and developing a plan to intervene. I became interested by reading some of the early articles published on the topic.

**Q. What are some of the challenges of working within dysphagia?**

**A.** It's one of the higher risk areas in which we work. If your evaluation is incorrect or your treatment not appropriate, not only may the patient fail to improve, but the patient's health status could decline. Conceivably, the patient might die from aspiration pneumonia.

**Q. How did you become more knowledgeable in dysphagia?**

**A.** Since dysphagia wasn't taught when I was in graduate school, I had to learn about the disorder through attending continuing education courses and reading everything I could get my hands on. I also collaborated with colleagues who were knowledgeable in the area.

**Q. What populations do clinicians usually work with within dysphagia?**

**A.** In the pediatric area, clinicians usually work with children who have a neurological disorder (e.g., cerebral palsy) or developmental delay that causes a swallowing/feeding problem. These children range in age from birth (when children are seen in the Neonatal Intensive Care Unit) through school-age. In the adult population, neurological disease and head and neck cancer are primary causes of dysphagia.

**Q. *What settings do clinicians work in?***

**A.** Dysphagia is treated in a variety of settings for both children and adults. Clinicians might work in a preschool, school, or in the child's home. They might see patients in a hospital, as an outpatient, in a rehabilitation facility, or through home health.

**Q. *What types of skills are needed to work in dysphagia that are not necessary for other specialty areas?***

**A.** Knowledge of neuroanatomy and neurophysiology, knowledge of the anatomy and physiology of the digestive track, and pulmonary function are necessary. Skill in performing and interpreting specific instrumental diagnostic procedures, such as a videofluoroscopic evaluation and endoscopic evaluation is necessary, as well as skill in working closely with a variety of other medical specialists.

**Q. *Are there any special kinds of certification necessary or available for dysphagia?***

**A.** The Certificate of Clinical Competence indicates that clinicians are ready to begin working independently with patients with dysphagia, if they have demonstrated competency to do so. Soon ASHA will offer Specialty Recognition in the area of swallowing and swallowing disorders. The Inaugural Board has determined what the requirements will be and will begin accepting applications soon. This will be a voluntary program and will not be required in order to work with patients with dysphagia.

**Q. *Are there any organizations that provide membership specifically for dysphagia?***

**A.** ASHA has Special Interest Division 13 for Swallowing and Swallowing Disorders. Students can join for a reduced fee. They will receive four newsletters a year with very informative articles. In addition, the Division has a listserve that is free to members of the Division. Students must be members of NSSLHA to join a Division.

**Q. *What are some good resources about dysphagia?***

**A.** The newsletters and listservs from the Special Interest Divisions are good resources. There is also an association called the Dysphagia Research Society, http://www.dysphagiaresearch.org, a multi-disciplinary society comprised of many different medical specialties and speech-language pathology. This society has a journal called *Dysphagia*.

**Q. *What are the best reasons to work within dysphagia?***

**A.** I think different aspects appeal to different people. Some of the reasons that I like working with patients with dysphagia are that there is often a quick improvement in their skills. Eating is such a fundamental part of our daily lives that a patient and their families are grateful when you can help the patient return to eating. In addition, it is an area that is gaining a strong evidence base; for instance, there is a lot of good research occurring in the area that supports what we do.

# VOICE
• • • • • • •

An interview with Diane Bless, Ph.D., CCC-SLP by Marie Patton, master's student, SLP, University of Wisconsin-Madison and NSSLHA president, 2001–2003. Dr. Bless is an ASHA Honors recipient who has done extensive research in voice. She is also a professor for voice disorders at the University of Wisconsin-Madison.

**Q. *What made you want to work within voice?***

**A.** There was not just one thing that led me to voice. I've always liked how voice represents a wide spectrum of ages and contexts. It's like a depth of a single field. Voice includes anatomy, physiology, drugs, physics, and singing. I like how you can make a significant difference in people's quality of life.

**Q. *What are some of the challenges of working within voice?***

**A.** The challenges are the same as what's exciting. You need to know so much and keep current in relevant areas, such as molecular biology.

**Q. *How did you become more knowledgeable in your specialty area?***

**A.** I started out volunteering. Later, I worked at clinics where I learned from clients who asked helpful and challenging questions. I had a post doctorate where I studied the larynx and voice in other fields outside of speech pathology.

**Q. *What populations (e.g., age ranges) do clinicians usually work with within voice?***

**A.** Clinicians work with infants up to geriatrics.

**Q. *Are there any specific settings that clinicians work within voice?***

**A.** Hospitals in the otolaryngology; speech pathology and neurology clinics; schools; theatrical environments; and computer programming environments with voice recognition systems and therapy material development.

**Q. *Are there any special kinds of certification necessary or available for voice?***

**A.** No, not specifically. The Denver Center for Performing Arts and the University of Iowa pair to create an intensive, twelve-week training program in voice. At the end of the training, participants receive a certificate. However, the experience is mostly about the educational aspects rather than receiving the certificate.

**Q.** *Are there any organizations that provide membership specifically for this specialty area?*

**A.** ASHA Special Interest Division 3: Voice and Voice Disorders has student affiliates. The Voice Foundation has student membership and membership includes the *Journal of Voice*. The American Academy of Otolaryngology (AAO), which gives students and students in their medical residency, reduced rates at meetings.

**Q.** *What are some conferences that are about voice?*

**A.** The Phonosurgery Conference in Madison, Wisconsin, takes place every even year. There's also the Voice Foundation Conference in Philadelphia. Speech-language pathologists, laryngologists, singers, voice coaches, patients, speech scientists, and engineers usually attend these conferences.

**Q.** *What types of skills are needed to work in voice that are not necessary for other areas?*

**A.** A firm foundation in structure and function in anatomy and physiology, how the psyche contributes to voice, and an understanding of how the human body works and apply that knowledge to treat a dysfunction.

Individuals who study voice have some of the following foci:

- Neurologically-based
- Psychologically-based
- Systemic problems (esophageal-based)
- Benign cancer
- Pathology on epithelial tissue

**Q.** *What are some good resources for voice?*

**A.** Books:

Aronson, A. (1990). *Clinical voice disorders: An interdisciplinary approach*. New York, NY: Thieme Medical Publishers.

Benninger, M. S., Jacobsen, B. H., & Johnson, A. F. (1994). *Vocal arts medicine: The care and prevention of professional voice disorders*. New York, NY: Thieme Medical Publishers.

Colton, R. H., & Casper, J. K. (1996). *Understanding voice problems*. Philadelphia, PA: Williams and Wilkins.

Fried, M. P. (1996). *The larynx: A multidisciplinary approach*. St. Louis, MO: Mosby.

Stemple, J. C. (2000). *Voice therapy: Clinical studies*. San Diego, CA: Singular/Thomson Delmar Learning.

Journals:

*The Journal of Voice*

All of the ASHA journals

*Advance*
*Journal of the Acoustical Society*
*Journal of Head and Neck Surgery*
*The Laryngescope*

**Q. What are the best reasons to work within voice?**

**A.** I cannot imagine another area being more rewarding. There's the people aspect where you can make a difference in fifteen minutes, or longer with people who have cancer or function problems. Treatment can include surgery and lasers. Plus, you can work with celebrities.

## CONCLUSION

If you find an interview to be particularly inspiring or one that fits with your professional goals, consider reading more about the specialty area, observing a clinician working with clients in these areas, requesting a clinical practicum in the area, and investigating whether your CSD program offers a course on the topic. If your program does not offer a course on the topic, consider having a directed study on the topic or look online for other universities that offer an online course. Also, search state and national associations' Web sites for upcoming continuing education events on the topic. Again, remember that this list of specialties is not exhaustive. If you think you are interested in something not listed here, speak with your professors to discuss additional areas to investigate.

# CHAPTER 27

## Other Career Options in CSD

### INTRODUCTION

Not all audiologists and speech-language pathologists remain clinicians throughout their careers. After practicing clinically for a period of time, some become professors and researchers, and others become administrators, such as assistant deans of CSD programs. Other options, not listed in the following interviews, include editor of a peer reviewed journal, clinical director, clinical supervisor, and school principal. If you start your career as a clinician and one day decide you would like to try something new, there will be plenty of career options available to you. This chapter provides interviews with professionals who have taken an alternate career path in CSD, and their experience may help you to have a more complete picture of the many opportunities you will have as a professional audiologist, speech-language pathologist, or speech/hearing scientist.

## PROFESSOR AND RESEARCHER

An interview with Brian Goldstein, Ph.D., CCC-SLP by Kelly Farquharson, NSSLHA Regional Councilor, Region I, 2003–2005. Dr. Goldstein is an Associate Professor at Temple University in Philadelphia, PA.

**Q. *What influenced you to become a university researcher?***

**A.** As an undergraduate linguistics major at Brandeis University, I realized that my knowledge of linguistics was (understandably) rather broad, but not very deep. Knowing a little about many things was frustrating to me. I felt the need to know about something in sufficient depth. For me, that "something" has always been phonology. Upon entering the master's program in speech-language pathology, I decided I would tailor my papers and assignments (when possible) to phonology, and Spanish phonology, in particular. So, in every class, I attempted to complete papers and very small research projects on aspects of Spanish phonology (e.g., my first paper in graduate school was a critique of phonological assessments designed for Spanish speakers). My interest in Spanish phonology and in research grew to the point that I completed my master's thesis on the use of phonological processes in typically developing Spanish-speaking

**193**

children (which was published in 1996 in *Language, Speech, and Hearing Services in the Schools*). When I completed the master's program, I decided I would pursue a doctorate at some point. I worked for two years as a staff SLP at Massachusetts General Hospital in Boston where about half my caseload was Spanish speaking. During those two years, I was able to complete two research studies that I presented at an ASHA convention. Increasingly, I began to envision a career in research and returned to Temple University for my Ph.D. Since my graduation, I have been actively involved in research.

**Q.** *What is your current area of research, and why do you think it is important to the field?*

**A.** My main research interest continues to be (almost 20 years after I started the master's program) Spanish phonological development and disorders. Currently, I am investigating how the phonological system may be represented in bilinguals. That is, are the phonological systems of both languages stored as one unit or are they stored separately? I think this research has both theoretical and clinical implications. Theoretically, it may begin to form the nature of bilingual (and perhaps even monolingual) phonological acquisition. Clinically, it will aid practicing SLPs in providing more appropriate assessment and intervention services to bilingual children.

**Q.** *What do you especially enjoy about being a researcher and instructor?*

**A.** Research is fun. One starts with a question in the field that needs to be answered. More often than not, that question starts as a clinical issue that needs to be solved; for example, in which languages(s) should bilingual children with speech and language disorders be treated? Then, you try to determine how to go about answering that question. So, I enjoy the process of going from question to method to results to theoretical and clinical implications. Usually the completion of one study necessitates another study to answer even more questions.

I also enjoy research because it is a collaborative process. I've never done any research all by myself; it always has involved other people. Research affords me the opportunity to discuss theoretical and practical issues with individuals who are interested in the same questions as I am.

Finally, I love research because I get to present it at conferences and then write it up to submit for publication in journals and book chapters. Being able to present research in a way that informs clinical practice is quite satisfying.

I have been involved in research for almost 20 years now. I do not regret one day of it. It's the best (professional) decision I ever made.

**Q.** *What are some of the challenges of working in research at a university?*

**A.** I think there are two main challenges in being a researcher at a university: time and resources. Research must be balanced with other university responsibilities, such as teaching, advising, and committee work. I don't see all these responsibilities as mutually exclusive, by the way. For example, I often use classes to present some of my own research to see how students react to my conclusions and clinical implications. Doing research is not only time intensive but also resource intensive. Thus, I am always trying to write grants to move along the research enterprise. Funds from grants can be used to support research assistants, pay participants, decrease teaching load, buy equipment and supplies, and fund travel to conferences to disseminate research results.

**Q.** *What types of skills/certification are needed to work in this specialty area that may not be necessary for other specialty areas?*

**A.** The two most important skills for a researcher are an independent drive and organizational skills (being reasonably intelligent and a quick study don't hurt either). These skills are clearly important for others in the field as well; however, they are paramount for researchers. An independent drive and organizational skills are critical, because when I am working on a research project, there is no one who "checks up on me" on a daily basis to make sure I am doing what I am supposed to be doing. I must be motivated and disciplined to do research without constant oversight. As I mentioned previously, research activities also must be balanced with other responsibilities. Being organized allows me to devote time to research, but also to prepare for class, advise master's and doctoral students, and work on committees in my department, in my university, and in organizations like ASHA.

**Q.** *Why, in your opinion, is it important for an SLP graduate student to consider research as a career option?*

**A.** Graduate students should consider research as a profession because it is a terrific career in a field in which researchers are desperately needed. Moreover, it affords a great deal of independence and flexibility. Through research, you are able to choose the topics you want to research, the questions you want to answer, the individuals you want to work with, and the venues where you would like to disseminate the information. The possibilities are endless.

In some way, graduate students are already researchers. Ultimately, they may not be producers of research (although it is my hope that many graduate students will get involved in some research in their master's program and after they graduate), but they are and will continue to be consumers of research. As you know, evidence-based practice is an important issue in our field right now. The evidence for efficacious and effective clinical approaches will come from on-going research activities. Graduate students may not be part of those studies, but they certainly will need to read them in the journals, understand them, and implement them in their day-to-day practice.

**Q. *What are some good resources for this specialty area? Are there any journals specific to this specialty area?***

**A.** The best resource for people interested in research is researchers themselves. Graduate students interested in research should not hesitate to go see faculty in their department who are active researchers. Students also should consider emailing prominent researchers and asking them about research opportunities. By and large, people in this field are approachable and would be more than happy to answer questions about the research process.

In addition, it is important to read the journals and make connections from the research to your daily practice. Depending on the research study, this is not always an easy task, but it is vital if the field is to continue to be taken seriously as one whose practice is built on a foundation of science.

# ASSISTANT DEAN

An interview with Ellen R. Cohn, Ph.D., CCC-SLP by Kelly Farquharson, NSSLHA Regional Councilor, Region I, 2003–2005. Dr. Cohn is Assistant Dean for the Instructional School of Health and Rehabilitation Sciences at the University of Pittsburgh. She is also an Associate Professor in the Department of Communication Science and Disorders, and former NSSLHA chapter advisor.

**Q. *How did you become an assistant dean?***

**A.** I did not seek the assistant dean position, but was appointed by our Dean following my service as the School's Director of Instructional Development. Prior to that, I had served as a university speech and hearing clinic director, and as our graduate program's clinical coordinator. When I look back, it is clear that my school positions emerged from serving on our Dean's committee to generate a strategic instructional technology plan, and as the elected secretary of our school faculty. I was also fortunate to receive excellent university-based exposure to teaching and instructional technology.

**Q. *What are some of your roles as an assistant dean?***

**A.** Each day is different! That's great, because I enjoy the variety of diverse, simultaneous challenges. A few of my responsibilities are to plan and organize faculty development programs, including our annual faculty retreat. I advise the Dean's Student Advisory Board, arrange for school events, and conduct student satisfaction surveys. New instructional programming is a key responsibility. Our faculty members and doctoral students frequently consult me concerning instruction, instructional technology, and issues related to academic integrity. I plan our Board of Visitors meetings, prepare the school's annual report and business plan, and author other documents as needed by our Dean. Deans of all levels usually serve on a lot of university committees, and I enjoy that as well. I also work closely with our school's development/public relations officer.

**Q. *What are some of the challenges of being an assistant dean?***

**A.** I currently balance 50% service in the dean's office with 50% commitment to my department. The greatest challenge is when the two schedules collide, and I need to be in two places at one time.

**Q. *What are some of the most rewarding aspects of being an assistant dean?***

**A.** It is a privilege to work with Dean Clifford Brubaker—as I constantly learn from him. Because he is a visionary leader, I've been included in innovative and remarkable programs, such as the McGowan Institute for Rehabilitation Medicine. It is delightful to interact with the many international visitors, national leaders in rehabilitation education and research, funders, and government officials who visit our school. Last year, I initiated a Masters of Law concentration in Disability Law at the University of Pittsburgh School of Law, which appears to be the first such program nationally. It is very rewarding when I can identify ways to initiate a new policy or practice that is helpful to my school community, and when I can directly assist students. I also enjoy the opportunity to nominate faculty and students for awards—especially when they win!

**Q. *Is there anything that students and young professionals can do now to make them an ideal candidate for becoming an assistant dean?***

**A.** Most assistant deans earn a Ph.D. and plan to spend their careers in academia. Become a good writer, editor, and public speaker. Learn all that you can about organizational communication and strategic planning. Become engaged in non-profit committees and boards, including NSSLHA, regional and state organizations, and United Way. Take advantage of every opportunity to upgrade your technology skills, and take an undergraduate course in human resources management. Enlarge your network so that you become conversant with other disciplines. The ASHA Special Interest Division 10: Issues in Higher Education, is a valuable resource. Always seek to work with great role models—persons who are leaders in their disciplines, generous mentors, ethical professionals, and who actively embrace the future.

# PUBLIC POLICY AND ASHA
# PRACTICE POLICY*

. . . . . . . . . . . . . . . . . . . . . . .

An interview with Arlene Pietranton, Ph.D., CCC-SLP by Marie Patton, master's student, SLP, University of Wisconsin-Madison and NSSLHA president, 2001–2003. Dr. Pietranton is currently the Executive Director of ASHA; a position she recently assumed after serving as the ASHA Chief Staff Officer for Speech-Language Pathology. Dr. Pietranton has also worked as the ASHA Director of Health Care Services, Administrative Director of the Neurological Institute at George Washington University (GWU) Medical Center, Director of Rehabilitation at GWU Medical Center, and Director of Speech-Language Pathology and Audiology at GWU.

**Q. *What made you want to work within the area of policy?***

**A.** I made a decision years ago to go into communication sciences and disorders because I wanted to help people. Along the way of providing services, I became a program director. I soon appreciated that overseeing programs was another important way of helping people. When I was in the field for about six years, I began to also realize that in delivering services, a lot of factors impact what services clinicians provide and how those services are reimbursed. I realized that there were people involved in making those "policy" decisions and I wanted to be one of the people who influenced their decisions.

**Q. *What did you do within the area of policy?***

**A.** Prior to becoming an ASHA staff member, I volunteered on ASHA committees, some that developed documents. I was occasionally among ASHA members invited to partner with ASHA staff who lobby. I represented the professions by attending meetings for what was then the Health Care Financing Administration (HCFA), and now is the Centers for Medicare and Medicaid Services (CMS). I also served on the ASHA Legislative Council, which makes decisions on what becomes ASHA policy. As a member of ASHA staff, I worked as an ex-officio member of several committees that developed policy documents, such as the Preferred Practice Patterns for Speech-Language Pathology and the 2001 SLP Scope of Practice. Since coming to the ASHA national office, I have done more work in public policy and ASHA policies. For example, when I was the Chief Staff Officer for Speech-Language Pathology, one program that reported to me was Government Relations and Public Policy (GRPP). I worked closely with the GRPP staff who lobby on behalf of ASHA and our professions.

---

*\*Public policies in CSD relate to the issues that the government adopted or is considering adopting that will affect professionals, students, and/or our clients. ASHA practice policies are the documents that ASHA members follow, such as position statements, knowledge and skills, and scope of practice.*

**Q. *What are some of the challenges of working within policy?***

**A.** In relation to public policy, there are two particular challenges. One, there's a need to educate the decision-makers, such as the members of congress and state education agencies, and those who need and receive our services. Two, advocating for a particular point of view can often be challenging because you will encounter people who have strong conflicting opinions from yours.

In ASHA policy making, a challenge, which is true for all clinical professions, is that there is a limited amount of strong research evidence of what is and is not effective in assessment and intervention approaches.

**Q. *When you first started working within policy, how did you become more knowledgeable in it?***

**A.** I'm a big believer in asking questions. There are always people around you who are knowledgeable, such as colleagues, friends, or ASHA staff. Be honest about what you know and don't know. Ask others for resources. Then be a good listener and reader.

**Q. *How can a person get involved in policy?***

**A.** For public and ASHA policy, you can be involved proactively and reactively. Proactively, you can periodically check the ASHA Web site on ASHA documents and advocacy. You can look up the current issues ASHA is advocating. Members can log on to a special section of the Web site, create a password, enter your zip code, and you'll get the mailing addresses and phone numbers of the legislators in your area. You can make a contribution to the ASHA Political Action Committee (PAC). You can be reactive to public and ASHA policy by responding to the notices that are available through listservs that you belong to, newsletters, and publications (e.g., NSSLHA *News and Notes, ASHA Leader*). For example, some ASHA listservs send out notices when a draft document is available for peer review.

Also, ASHA's annual public policy agenda is on the ASHA Web site. The agenda is developed by the GRPP board. They send emails and other messages out to ASHA and NSSLHA members and ask what issues they would like to see addressed on the GRPP agenda.

What strikes me is the opportunities for clinicians, students, and those in academe to be aware of and involved in the public policy and ASHA policy. Before the mid-90s when the internet exploded, the main opportunity for involvement was through the mail. Members would provide a peer review by writing comments by hand and mailing them into ASHA. Now policies, peer reviews, and public policies are posted on the Web, emails are sent out with the ASHA link, and the *ASHA Leader* has postings. The availability of the policies is just tremendous. It is much easier to be involved now than it was 15 to 20 years ago.

**Q.** *What types of skills are needed to work in policy?*

**A.** You need to be committed to your profession, have a passion for what you do, know how important the field is to those who receive your services, and know how the decisions that are made by others impact those services. You also need good communication skills. You should be able to step back and see other people's perspectives and respect them. Good advocates can see how the other party looks at things, and use that knowledge to help the other party to see their viewpoint. Finally, you need to be persistent.

**Q.** *What are some good resources for students who are just getting started in learning more about policy?*

**A.** For public policy, the ASHA Web site has a lot of good information on the current issues, how to make a Hill visit, and how to connect with members of congress.

For ASHA policy on the Web site, you can read about ASHA governance. You can find out individuals' names who serve on the ASHA Executive Board, Legislative Council or a committee or board and contact them with your concerns.

**Q.** *What are the best reasons to be involved in policy?*

**A.** Policy decisions will have an impact on who will receive your services, what services will be reimbursed, and define what is best practice. By being involved, you can help assure that good policy decisions are made.


## CONCLUSION

This chapter is just a brief introduction to the communication sciences and disorders career options that exist outside of clinical work. If you know that you are interested in pursuing one of these tracks, consider interviewing individuals in these jobs to find out what you can do to prepare yourself. Do not stop with just the options listed herein; talk with other professionals in the field, your professors, and peers to uncover all the opportunities that may be out there waiting for you.

# CHAPTER 28

# Resumé and Interview Preparation

Lee Cruz, Assistant Director of Placement Services, Counseling and
Career Services, Saint Xavier University

## INTRODUCTION

Now that you have mastered your academic coursework and will soon graduate (if
you have not already), it is time to stake your claim in a professional position. This
chapter provides an overview of what you need to know to get a job as an audiologist or speech-language pathologist. It also provides a number of excellent
resources, such as sample letters, a sample resumé, and other documents to use in
your job search. Just as with applications to degree programs, the more research
you do to find the right types of jobs, and the more preparation you put into your
resumé, letters, and other materials, the greater your chances of getting the job that
fulfills your personal aspirations.

## RESUMÉ WRITING

The resumé is intended to secure the interview, which in turn, is intended to
secure the position. It should concisely highlight your career goals, educational
background, work experiences, special skills, accomplishments, and activities
in a manner that will market you effectively. Figures 28-1, 28-2, and 28-3 are
three examples of formats to consider when preparing your resumé. Following
are the essential elements to any resumé.

### Heading

The heading, usually listed at the top of your resumé, assures that employers
can call, mail, or email you with relative ease. Avoid listing a work number,
because it is often awkward or difficult for a potential employer to contact you
at a place of employment. Make certain that your email address sounds professional; snuggly_wuggly@email.com or partymonster78@email.com really are
not going to make a great first impression to a potential employer.

---

**Kerry J. Doe**

123 State Road • Orland Park, Illinois 60462
(708) 555-1111 • kdoe@mailbox.com

**OBJECTIVE**
To obtain a speech-language pathologist clinical fellowship position in an education cooperative.

**EDUCATION**
*XYZ University – New Lenox, Illinois*
**Master of Science: Speech-Language Pathology**
    Graduation Date: May 2003, GPA: 3.9/4.0
**Bachelor of Science: Speech-Language Pathology**
    Graduation Date: May 2000, GPA: 3.8/4.0 (Magna Cum Laude)

**CERTIFICATION**
Illinois Type 03/09 Certificate in Speech and Language Pathology – May, 2003
Illinois Test of Certification for Speech and Language Impaired – April, 2003
National Examination of Speech-Language Pathology and Audiology – April, 2003

**SKILLS**
Fluent in English and Polish languages, both verbal and written.

**PRESENTATIONS**
"New Trends in Speech Therapy for the Adolescent Down Syndrome Client"
• PowerPoint presentation conducted at the Associated Colleges of the Chicagoland Area Conference, March, 2002.

**RELEVANT EXPERIENCE**
*Wainwright Elementary School – Minooka, Illinois*
**Speech-Language Pathology Assistant (8/00–5/01)**
• Provided one-on-one instruction to Kindergarten students requiring speech and language therapy.
• Implemented therapies designed by the school's speech-language therapist.
• Contributed to planning sessions at multi-disciplinary committee meetings.

**CLINICAL EXPERIENCE**
*Green Point Elementary School – Palos Park, Illinois*
**Graduate Student Teacher (1/03–5/03)**
• Conducted assessments and developed individual education plans for students with communication deficiencies such as dysphagia, stuttering, language delays, and articulation and phonological disorders.
• Incorporated modern technologies to assist cross-categorical students with communication disorders.
• Met with family members to discuss clients' progress and to establish future goals and objectives.
• Participated in Student Services team meetings and multi-disciplinary conferences to discuss caseloads.
• Conducted a seminar for classroom teachers on ways to detect possible speech-language disorders.

*(continues)*

**Figure 28-1**    Resumé sample 1

## Kerry J. Doe - page 2

*Claybough Rehabilitation Center - Oak Lawn, Illinois*
**Graduate Practicum Hospital Clinician (8/02–12/02)**
- Performed evaluations and developed appropriate goals and objectives for elderly clients with communication disorders such as aphasia, right hemisphere dysfunction, and traumatic brain injury.
- Worked extensively with elderly dysphagia clients, including regulating diets to avoid aspiration.
- Collaborated with occupational and physical therapy teams to provide treatments for clients.
- Acquired comprehensive knowledge of videofluoroscopy assessment instrumentation.
- Maintained accurate comprehensive records of clients' therapy sessions.

*Smith Speech and Language Clinic, XYZ University - New Lenox, Illinois*
**Graduate Student Clinician (8/01–5/02)**
- Conducted assessments and established appropriate therapies for children, ages 5–12, with a wide variety of communication disorders in articulation, language, auditory processing, and fluency.
- Convened with parents to discuss children's development and further therapy goals and objectives.

**Undergraduate Student Clinician (1/00–5/00)**
- Developed and implemented individual treatment plans for clients with communication disorders, including apraxia, language delays, and articulation and phonological disorders.

**HONORS**
Knudsen-Kempton Graduate Student Leadership Award, 2002
Speech-Language Pathology Senior Student of the Year Award, 2000

**MEMBERSHIPS**
National Student Speech-Language-Hearing Association (NSSLHA)
Illinois Speech-Language-Hearing Association (ISHA)

**ACTIVITIES**
Speech Club, XYZ University
- Communications Chairperson, 2001–02
- Coordinated a mentoring program for undergraduate speech-language pathology majors.

### References Available Upon Request

**Figure 28-1** (Continued)

---

**Kerry J. Doe**
123 State Road • Orland Park, Illinois 60462
(708) 555-1111 • kdoe@mailbox.com

---

**Objective**
To obtain a speech-language pathologist clinical fellowship position in an education cooperative.

**Education**
**XYZ University,** New Lenox, Illinois
Master of Science: *Speech-Language Pathology*
Graduation Date: May, 2003, GPA: 3.9/4.0

Bachelor of Science: *Speech-Language Pathology*
Graduation Date: May, 2000, GPA: 3.8/4.0 (Magna Cum Laude)

**Certification**
Illinois Type 03/09 Certificate in Speech and Language Pathology – May, 2003
Illinois Test of Certification for Speech and Language Impaired – April, 2003
National Examination of Speech-Language Pathology and Audiology – April, 2003

**Skills**
Fluent in English and Polish languages, both verbal and written.

**Presentations**
"New Trends in Speech Therapy for the Adolescent Down Syndrome Client"
• PowerPoint presentation conducted at the Associated Colleges of the Chicagoland Area Conference, March, 2002.

**Relevant Experience**
**Wainwright Elementary School,** Minooka, Illinois
*Speech-Language Pathology Assistant* (8/00–5/01)
• Provided one-on-one instruction to Kindergarten students requiring speech and language therapy.
• Implemented therapies designed by the school's speech-language therapist.
• Contributed to planning sessions at multi-disciplinary committee meetings.

**Clinical Experience**
**Green Point Elementary School,** Palos Park, Illinois
*Graduate Student Teacher* (1/03–5/03)
• Conducted assessments and developed individual education plans for students with communication deficiencies such as dysphagia, stuttering, language delays, and articulation and phonological disorders.
• Incorporated modern technologies to assist cross-categorical students with communication disorders.
• Met with family members to discuss clients' progress and to establish future goals and objectives.

*(continues)*

**Figure 28-2** Resumé sample 2

**Kerry J. Doe - page 2**

- Participated in Student Services team meetings and multi-disciplinary conferences to discuss caseloads.
- Conducted a seminar for classroom teachers on ways to detect possible speech-language disorders.

**Claybough Rehabilitation Center,** Oak Lawn, Illinois
*Graduate Practicum Hospital Clinician* (8/02–12/02)
- Performed evaluations and developed appropriate goals and objectives for elderly clients with communication disorders such as aphasia, right hemisphere dysfunction, and traumatic brain injury.
- Worked extensively with elderly dysphagia clients, including regulating diets to avoid aspiration.
- Collaborated with occupational and physical therapy teams to provide treatments for clients.
- Acquired comprehensive knowledge of videofluoroscopy assessment instrumentation.
- Maintained accurate comprehensive records of clients' therapy sessions.

**Smith Speech and Language Clinic, XYZ University,** New Lenox, Illinois
*Graduate Student Clinician* (8/01–5/02)
- Conducted assessments and established appropriate therapies for children, ages 5–12, with a wide variety of communication disorders in articulation, language, auditory processing, and fluency.
- Convened with parents to discuss children's development and further therapy goals and objectives.

*Undergraduate Student Clinician* (1/00–5/00)
- Developed and implemented individual treatment plans for clients with communication disorders, including apraxia, language delays, and articulation and phonological disorders.

**Honors**
Knudsen-Kempton Graduate Student Leadership Award, 2002
Speech-Language Pathology Senior Student of the Year Award, 2000

**Memberships**
National Student Speech-Language-Hearing Association (NSSLHA)
Illinois Speech-Language-Hearing Association (ISHA)

**Activities**
Speech Club, XYZ University
- Communications Chairperson, 2001–02
- Coordinated a mentoring program for undergraduate speech-language pathology majors.

**References Available Upon Request**

**Figure 28-2** (Continued)

## Kerry J. Doe

123 State Road • Orland Park, Illinois 60462 • (708) 555-1111 • kdoe@mailbox.com

**OBJECTIVE**
To obtain a speech-language pathologist clinical fellowship position in an education cooperative.

**EDUCATION**
*XYZ University – New Lenox, Illinois*
**Master of Science: Speech-Language Pathology**
Graduation Date: May, 2003, GPA: 3.9/4.0

**Bachelor of Science: Communication Sciences and Disorders**
Graduation Date: May, 2000, GPA: 3.8/4.0 (Magna Cum Laude)

**CERTIFICATION**
Illinois Type 03/09 Certificate in Speech and Language Pathology – May, 2003
Illinois Test of Certification for Speech and Language Impaired – April, 2003
National Examination of Speech-Language Pathology and Audiology – April, 2003

**MEMBERSHIPS**
National Student Speech-Language-Hearing Association (NSSLHA)
Illinois Speech-Language-Hearing Association (ISHA)

**RELEVANT EXPERIENCE**
*Wainwright Elementary School – Minooka, Illinois*
**Speech-Language Pathology Assistant** (8/00–5/01)
• Provided one-on-one instruction to Kindergarten students requiring speech and language therapy.
• Implemented therapies designed by the school's speech-language therapist.
• Contributed to planning sessions at multi-disciplinary committee meetings.

**CLINICAL EXPERIENCE**
*Green Point Elementary School – Palos Park, Illinois*
**Graduate Student Teacher** (1/03–5/03)
• Conducted assessments and developed individual education plans for students with communication deficiencies such as dysphagia, stuttering, language delays, and articulation and phonological disorders.
• Incorporated modern technologies to assist cross-categorical students with communication disorders.
• Met with family members to discuss clients' progress and to establish future goals and objectives.

*(continues)*

**Figure 28-3**  Resumé sample 3

**Kerry J. Doe - page 2**

- Participated in Student Services team meetings and multi-disciplinary conferences to discuss caseloads.
- Conducted a seminar for classroom teachers on ways to detect possible speech-language disorders.

*Claybough Rehabilitation Center – Oak Lawn, Illinois*
**Graduate Practicum Hospital Clinician** (8/02–12/02)
- Performed evaluations and developed appropriate goals and objectives for elderly clients with communication disorders such as aphasia, right hemisphere dysfunction, and traumatic brain injury.
- Worked extensively with elderly dysphagia clients, including regulating diets to avoid aspiration.
- Collaborated with occupational and physical therapy teams to provide treatments for clients.
- Acquired comprehensive knowledge of videofluoroscopy assessment instrumentation.
- Maintained accurate comprehensive records of clients' therapy sessions.

*Smith Speech and Language Clinic, XYZ University – New Lenox, Illinois*
**Graduate Student Clinician** (8/01–5/02)
- Conducted assessments and established appropriate therapies for children, ages 5–12, with a wide variety of communication disorders in articulation, language, auditory processing, and fluency.
- Convened with parents to discuss children's development and further therapy goals and objectives.

**Undergraduate Student Clinician** (1/00–5/00)
- Developed and implemented individual treatment plans for clients with communication disorders, including apraxia, language delays, and articulation and phonological disorders.

**References Available Upon Request**

**Figure 28-3** (Continued)

## Objective

Your career objective should be succinct and should show career focus, possibly emphasizing a couple of your strongest skills. You can always change it to fit a particular position. Avoid using personal pronouns (I, me, my). Listing an objectve is important for resumés of individuals who may not have much professional work experience. You may, however, find that individuals who have been working for a long time delete this feature. Until you have a number of years of professional experience under your belt, the objective is important to your resumé.

## Education

List only your college/graduate education, placing your most recent school first and working backwards chronologically. Include any degree earned, major, minor, and graduation date. Listing your grade point average is optional but recommended, especially if it is at least a 3.0 on a 4.0 scale. Indicate what kind of maximum grading scale was used at that institution.

## Certification

List any certifications that you have attained, as well as licensing examinations that you are scheduled to take. You may mention the dates associated with those items.

## Honors

Indicate any scholarships, awards, or honors earned during your college career, including special graduation honors, membership to any honor societies, or awards such as Dean's List.

## Activities

These are good indicators of your leadership, professional interests, contributions, and social skills. Include those affiliations of which you are/were a member at school and/or in your community. List the offices that you held with those organizations. If applicable, mention highlights of accomplishments that you have achieved in those organizations. If you prefer, you may list the dates that you were associated with those activities. Avoid listing those associations that have a radical or harsh political or social tone to them, because prospective employers may perceive that you have extreme, inflexible convictions. Often employers are looking to get a strong picture of you as a person, and the activities you list are one way they get to know "who" you are.

# Presentations

List any out-of-class presentations that you have conducted, including where and when they were performed. This is where you would list any poster sessions or other presentations at conferences, such as the annual ASHA Convention.

# Skills

Mention any special abilities that you possess, such as computer proficiencies, instrumentation competencies, or foreign language fluencies.

# Experience

List your experiences in reverse chronological order. Include full-time jobs, part-time jobs, co-ops, internships, volunteer jobs, clinicals, practicums, field experiences, etc. List organization names, cities, states, dates of employment, job titles, responsibilities, and accomplishments. Use action words to describe your responsibilities and achievements, and be cautious to use the correct verb tense. Create phrases that are brief, but make them meaningful and at least five words long. List items that highlight relevant skills, special training, high-level accountability, and achievement. If applicable, mention quantitative illustrations of contributions and accomplishments. When listing your responsibilities, use aligned bullet points instead of a paragraph format.

# References

A simple overall statement will suffice (e.g., References available upon request.). However, you probably should have a set of references ready on a separate page, in case they are requested. You should have at least three professional references that speak of your work ethic objectively, such as current or former supervisors or instructors. It is common courtesy to ask permission before listing someone as a reference. List names, job titles, company names, addresses, telephone numbers, and email addresses. Figure 28-4 is an example of a standard reference page.

# Miscellaneous

If you need to include some information not applicable to any of previous sections, list another heading (e.g., Clinical Experiences, Publications, Presentations, Licenses, Certifications, Additional Training, Professional Development, Conferences, Seminars, Workshops). Arrange the sections in the order that markets you best, with your greatest selling points ideally in the upper two-thirds of the document. Make certain that your section headings are distinct.

# Kerry J. Doe

### References

**Mary Jones**
*Speech Pathologist/Clinical Supervisor*
Harrison Elementary School
579 W. Main Street
Mokena, IL 60448
(708) 555-7777
mjones@dist157.org

**James Meyer**
*Audiology Professor*
ABC University
1 E. Wire Drive
Frankfort, IL 60423
(815) 555-2222
jmeyer@abcuniv.edu

**John Smith**
*Speech-Language Pathology Professor*
ABC University
1 E. Wire Drive
Frankfort, IL 60423
(815) 555-3333
jsmith@abcuniv.edu

**Patricia Washington**
*Audiology Professor*
ABC University
1 E. Wire Drive
Frankfort, IL 60423
(815) 555-4444
pwashington@abcuniv.edu

**Michael Williams**
*Special Education Resource Teacher*
Harrison Elementary School
579 W. Main Street
Mokena, IL 60448
(708) 555-8888
mwilliams@dist157.org

**Figure 28-4** References

Use italics, boldfacing, and bullets to add variety and to place emphasis in certain areas, but do not overuse them to the point that your resumé looks too busy. Keep the content and formatting consistent. Use page margins of about .4- to .5-inch for the top and bottom, with .7- to 1.0-inch for the left and right sides. For ease of readability, always use a computer, an 11- or 12-point font size, a basic font type, and a laser printer. Copy your resumé onto high quality paper of a neutral color, such as light gray or cream. An employer typically reviews a resumé initially for only a minute or two, so it is important to thoroughly sell your skills and experience in a succinct way.

Always proofread (repeatedly!) your resumé to ensure accuracy and consistency. Have a friend proofread for grammar, punctuation, and consistency in your spacing around bullets or other features of your resumé. Make sure that if you use a period after one description of a job, you use a period after every description of a job. Employers really do weed out undesirable candidates based on mistakes on the resumé.

## GUIDELINES FOR WRITING COVER LETTERS

A cover letter is the professional letter that accompanies your resumé, and can also be called an application letter or letter of interest. This section discusses the requirements for a cover letter.

### Format

A professionally styled cover letter utilizes a block format to give it a clean appearance. All the sections should be typed in single space format, with double spacing used only to separate the sections. Figure 28-5 is an example of a common format used for cover letters.

### Heading

The heading should list your address, telephone number, and the date. The next section includes the recruiter's name, his or her job title, the organization's name, and its address. The salutation should be formal and directed to a specific individual, whenever possible. If there is no way of ascertaining a specific addressee, then use the greeting "Dear Administrator:", "Dear Employer:", or "Dear Recruiter:", not "Dear Madam or Sir:" or "To Whom It May Concern:".

### Opening Paragraph

Name the specific position or type of work for which you are applying, and indicate from which resource (Web site, career center, newspaper, employee, instructor, etc.) you learned of the opening or organization.

---

**Kerry J. Doe**

123 State Road • Orland Park, Illinois 60462 • (708) 555-1111 • kdoe@mailbox.com

May 29, 2004

Melissa Smith
Assistant Superintendent
Fairview School District 123
7890 W. Main Street
Fairview, IL 61432

Dear Ms. Smith:

Please accept the enclosed resumé in consideration for the Speech Therapist-Clinical Fellowship position that is currently advertised on your Web site. I recently completed my graduate studies and am eager to start my career with your school district.

In addition to a master's degree in speech-language pathology and its accompanying clinical experiences, my background includes a year of **experience as a Speech Assistant** in an educational setting. All of those endeavors have allowed me to work with a wide range of clients, assessment tools, and therapies. They have also greatly enhanced my **analytical** and **goal setting skills**, and have significantly increased my awareness of the qualities necessary to be a successful speech therapist. My **creative** and **enthusiastic** approach to instruction enables me to quickly secure clients' interest, which allows me to provide for a positive learning experience. In addition, my effective **listening** and **communication skills**, along with my strong sense of **patience**, tend to gain clients' trust in my commitment to their well-being. Furthermore, my solid qualities of **resourcefulness** and **perseverance** help me to earn respect from clients and colleagues alike. Thus, my experience and personal characteristics seem to make me a suitable match for a career in speech-language pathology.

I would appreciate the opportunity to meet with you to discuss my qualifications in detail. Please send me any materials needed to complete the application process. If you have any questions or wish to arrange an interview, please feel free to contact me at your convenience at (708) 555-1111. Thank you very much for your valuable time and consideration.

**Sincerely,**

*Kerry Doe*
Kerry Doe

**Figure 28-5** Cover letter example

# Middle Paragraph(s)

Indicate the reasons you are interested in and qualified for the position. Explain how your skills, academic background, work experiences, practicums, clinicals, internships, co-ops, and activities make you a well-suited candidate for the position. Refer to the specific achievements or unique qualifications you acquired in those experiences. Review the requirements for the position, and then try to match them with concrete examples that prove you actually possess those skills. Mention something about the organization that motivates you to want to work for it. Avoid repeating exactly the same information the reader will find on your resumé.

# Closing Paragraph

State your desire for a personal interview. Repeat your telephone number and email address, and offer any assistance to help in a speedy response. Finally, finish with a statement that will encourage a response, such as "I look forward to hearing from you," or "I look forward to speaking with you further about my qualifications."

# Ending

The ending should simply read "Sincerely," or "Yours truly," with your name typed three or four lines down to allow ample space for your signature above it.

# Miscellaneous

Limit your document to one page. Although it is okay to use the personal pronoun "I," avoid using it too frequently. While still sounding professional and somewhat formal, try to use common language to sound natural. Review the letter carefully, since the reader will probably perceive it to be an example of your written communication skills. Print it on the same type of paper that you use for your resumé.

Just as you proofread your resumé, proofread your cover letter. A prospective employer may not even bother to read your resumé if your cover letter has errors. Consider asking a friend to look it over for punctuation and spelling mistakes, as well as clarity and readability. This is your prospective employer's first glimpse of who you are. An unprofessional cover letter may mean it is also the last.

# INTERVIEW SKILLS

In an interview, an employer is ultimately looking to determine whether or not you have the necessary skills and experience to fill the position, as well as the type of personality that will connect with others affiliated with the organization. The following steps will help prepare you for the interview process.

# Before the Interview

***Do a Self-Assessment.*** Determine your short- and long-range career goals. Identify your skills, abilities, personal qualities, strengths, weaknesses, values, and interests. Determine how they fit the position for which you are applying. Be able to cite concrete examples of how you have demonstrated all those intangibles. Use your experiences from classes, internships, extracurricular activities, volunteer experiences, and work experiences to extract those examples. Focus on your accomplishments whenever possible. Be prepared to explain the rewards and satisfactions of your career field that caused you to choose it. Recruiters tend to shy away from candidates who have merely stumbled into their profession without much thought.

***Research the Organization.*** It is essential to know some detailed information about the company and the position prior to the interview. An interviewer may be reluctant to consider a candidate who does not commit time to previewing the organization or the position. Organization research also helps you to devise insightful responses and thought-provoking questions for an interview. Research the organization's mission, products and services, target markets, competitors, business strategies, future plans, challenges, and factors and trends affecting the industry. You can obtain this information through the Internet, libraries, chambers of commerce, directories, and individual organization literature.

***Prepare for Both Traditional and Behavioral-Based Questions.*** Some recruiters use the traditional method, in which they ask about your opinions and experiences on certain work-related issues. Others use the behavioral-based format, in which they question you about past situations and what you did under those conditions. The premise of the latter is that your past actions may be indicators of your future behaviors. Be ready to discuss the kinds of leadership, teamwork, initiative, planning, and organization you demonstrated for a given situation. Talk about the scenario, your course of action, the result, and what you learned from the experience. Be honest, but make certain to relay an account that reflects positively on you. Figure 28-6 contains examples of some common interview questions.

***Dress Professionally.*** The first impression that you make on an interviewer is your personal appearance. Improper attire can distract from anything positive that you convey about yourself during the interview. A traditional, conservative look is usually your safest bet.

- *Wardrobe Suggestions for Women:* Pant suits and skirt suits with hemlines that fall just below the knee are preferred. A navy blue, gray, or charcoal suit with a white, long-sleeved, cotton or silk blouse is recommended. Shoes should be black, brown, or navy, with a heel height that is comfortable for walking. Hosiery should be a neutral shade. Jewelry should be limited to one pair of simple earrings, a necklace, watch, and wedding band.

- Tell me about yourself.
- Tell me about your relevant experience/clinical practicum.
- What did you like best/worst about your clinical experiences?
- What types of assessments/therapies do you feel comfortable administering?
- In what area do you think you need the most training/supervision?
- How would you implement an IEP?
- How would you keep track of client progress?
- How do you work with a patient who is making very little progress?
- How do you determine whether or not your service for a client is successful?
- What expectations do you have of your clients? Of their parents/ family?
- How would you work with parents/family members of clients enrolled in your program?
- How would you relate your intervention to a client's classroom work?
- How would you handle a client who is openly frustrated and gives up?
- What types of professional conferences/workshops have you attended/are interested in attending?
- Would you feel comfortable presenting an in-service workshop to teachers, social workers, or nurses?
- Why did you choose speech-language pathology as a career?
- What do you find rewarding about this field?
- What do you consider to be your greatest strengths and weaknesses?
- What are your short-term and long-range career goals?
- What three characteristics describe you best?
- What are your three greatest accomplishments? ① School
- Why should I hire you? ② Artic clinic
- How would you describe the ideal job for you? ③

*(continues)*

**Figure 28-6** Interview questions

- What qualities should a successful speech-language pathologist possess?

- What qualities should a good supervisor possess?

- What type of relationship would you like to establish with your supervisor?

- What kind of work environment/management style do you prefer?

- How has your education prepared you for a career in speech-language pathology?

- Describe your most rewarding academic experience.

- Why did you select your college or university?

- Do you think that your grades are a good indication of your ability level?

- How do you think you can make a meaningful contribution to our organization?

- Why do you want to work for this organization?

- What do you know about our organization?

- Describe a major problem you encountered and how you dealt with it.

- Describe a time when you failed to meet expectations on an assignment.

- Describe a time when someone criticized your work in front of others and your reaction to it.

- Describe a negative situation when it was important for you to maintain a positive attitude.

- Describe a time when you had to deal with a difficult person (client, classmate, co-worker, etc.).

- Describe a time when you got co-workers or classmates of dissimilar backgrounds, interests, or goals to collaborate productively on a project.

**Questions to Ask an Employer at an Interview**

- What are some of the therapy objectives you would like accomplished?

- What would my typical day entail?

*(continues)*

**Figure 28-6** (Continued)

- What qualities are you looking for in candidates for this position?

- What characteristics do successful employees of this organization seem to have in common?

- Do you encourage attendance at certain conferences, workshops, and other educational activities?

- How often are performance reviews given?

- How is one evaluated?

- What do you like best about your job? This organization?

- What are some of the more difficult challenges someone in this position tends to encounter?

- Who determines the size and composition of my caseload?

- What kind of equipment/instruments/resources do you have?

- Would you please describe typical client in this program?

- What is the next course of action? When should I expect to hear from you?

*Sources:* American Speech-Language-Hearing Association, 2003; *Opportunities in Speech-Language Pathology Careers*, 2002

**Figure 28-6** (Continued)

Hairstyle should look controlled. Make-up should achieve a natural look, and nail polish should be conservative and neat. Avoid overwhelming perfumes. Keep all tattoos covered, if possible.

- *Wardrobe Suggestions for Men:* A two-piece, single-breasted navy blue, gray, or charcoal suit with a white, cotton, long-sleeved shirt is preferred. The tie should complement the suit and should not be too "loud." Shoes should be black or brown leather and polished, with socks that complement the suit. Jewelry should be limited to a wedding band and a watch, and all earrings should be removed. Hair should be well-groomed, and facial hair should be trimmed neatly. Avoid overbearing cologne or aftershave. Keep all tattoos covered, if possible.

*Be Organized.* You should arrive at least 15 to 20 minutes prior to the scheduled interview time. Allot yourself plenty of time to accommodate for getting lost, being stalled by construction, getting stuck in traffic, or having difficulty finding a parking space or the interview room. If necessary, consult an online map to gauge the distance and directions to your destination. You may be required to fill out an application before the interview, so bring addresses and telephone numbers of previous employers, professional references, and personal references. Bring extra copies of your resumé. Carry all those materials in a vinyl- or leather-bound folder, along with a couple of pens. Be courteous to everybody at the facility, regardless of their relationship to your interview.

## During the Interview

***Be Aware of Your Non-Verbal Communication.*** Always start with a smile and a firm handshake. Those simple gestures convey your level of self-confidence and are indicators of how proficient your interpersonal skills may be. Relax, maintain good eye contact, and keep your posture controlled. Interviewers are aware that you may be nervous, but it should not be acutely obvious. Deliver your answers with a sense of energy. Organizations need employees who have a personable and enthusiastic presence.

***Speak in a Clear, Articulate, Specific Manner.*** This is not the time to be shy and reticent. At the same time, avoid rambling, discursive speeches. Take your time and think about your answers before communicating them. Recruiters are seeking resourceful, effective communicators who can summon up logical, rational responses to a wide variety of professional issues. Be able to succinctly show how you fit the position and the organization's climate. Give specific examples that demonstrate how your strengths fit the characteristics that are required of the position. Confidently assert the reasons you are a valuable asset to your chosen profession. Stay sincere, because it is very difficult to keep track of lies and even harder to live up to them on the job.

***Remain Positive.*** Show motivation and enthusiasm by explaining why you want the position. Be ready to identify the positive qualities you can bring to the organization. Avoid debasing a former employer or talking negatively about a past work experience. If you are asked to discuss a negative experience, relay how you turned it into a positive one and what you learned from it. Employers are looking for candidates who maintain a positive attitude and a team spirit during even adverse times.

***Refer to Sample Items.*** Consider bringing a portfolio containing samples of your project work, recommendation letters, thank you letters received, awards, congratulatory letters, and/or performance evaluations. Refer to those samples when you are attempting to demonstrate something you mention. If you do use them, make certain you have copies of everything, in case an employer wants to hold on to some for review.

**Close Effectively.** Closing effectively means ending the interview with well-thought out questions. Questions indicate interest and show that you have actually given the position much thought. Figure 28-6 also contains some examples of questions that you may consider asking the employer. Do not inquire about salary and benefits. The employer will divulge these eventually, although maybe not until after an offer is made. Asking about salary conveys that you are more interested in the money than you are in the opportunity. Briefly summarize with some basic statements about how your aptitude and abilities fit in with the position. Ask what the next course of action is. Request business cards from your interviewers, and thank everyone for their time.

## After the Interview

**Send Thank You Letters.** Thank you letters are not optional; they are essential and employers expect them. They should be mailed within 24 hours after the interview. You can type or email your thank you letter. Thank you letters indicate that you are cordial and that you are grateful for the opportunity to interview. They also display your enthusiasm for the position you are seeking to attain. Thank everybody for the chance to interview, reminding them about the specific position for which you applied. The business cards you requested at the conclusion of each interview will be helpful when you are writing your thank you letters. Reiterate your interest in the position and the organization, and mention the skills and qualities you can bring to the company that make you an ideal candidate for the position. Figure 28-7 is an example of a thank you letter to an employer. The following suggestions can be used to create an effective thank you letter.

- *First Paragraph:* Thank the interviewer for the opportunity to meet with them, stating the position for which you interviewed and the date of the interview.

- *Second Paragraph:* Re-emphasize how your skills and experiences might make you an ideal match for the position, mentioning something that is especially appealing.

- *Third Paragraph:* Reaffirm your interest in the position and the organization. State your willingness to provide additional information. Thank all interviewers for their time and consideration.

## JOB SEARCH RESOURCES
• • • • • • • • • • • • • • • • • • • • • • • • • • • • • • • •

Not sure where to start your employment search? Try these resources:

- Directories of special education cooperatives/joint agreements

- Directories of public schools at http://www.ed.gov

- Directories of human care services

---

**Kerry J. Doe**

123 State Road • Orland Park, Illinois 60462 • (708) 555-1111 • kdoe@mailbox.com

March 10, 2004

Melissa Smith
Assistant Superintendent
Fairview School District 123
7890 W. Main Street
Fairview, IL 61432

Dear Ms. Smith:

Thank you very much for interviewing me for the Speech Therapist-Clinical Fellowship position with your school district today. You and your colleagues provided me with a very warm reception and informative discussion.

My enthusiasm for working with your district was strengthened as a result of our meeting, and the opportunity is congruent with the type of experience I am seeking. As mentioned during our conversation, my experiences as a Speech Assistant and as a Student Clinician have prepared me extensively for the type of work required of a Speech Pathologist in a school environment. In addition, my positive interpersonal qualities, proficient analytical abilities, and strong communication skills would make me an ideal candidate for the position. Furthermore, my willingness to assist with your college mentoring program would enable me to be a versatile contributor to your organization.

Once again, I wish to reiterate my genuine interest in the position and your organization. If you have any questions, please contact me at 708-555-1111. Thank you very much for your valuable time and consideration.

Sincerely,

*Kerry Doe*

Kerry Doe

---

**Figure 28-7** Thank you letter

- ASHA Career Center/Placement Center at http://www.asha.org
- Job fairs (especially education and health care career fairs)
- College/university career center job listings
- Sunday newspaper classified ads
- Professional associations
- Networking
- Web pages

## CONCLUSION

Now that you have almost completed (or have completed) your course of study, it would be nice if there were a great job just waiting for you. Unfortunately, it is not quite as easy as that. Sometimes things work out that a person gets the first job he or she applies for, but applying for jobs can often feel like a full-time job in itself, and it may take repeated interviews and a good amount of time before the right position is found. Be prepared to put in the time to first find jobs that are suited to your needs and interests, and then to create high-quality, error-free documents like your resumé, cover letter, and thank you letter. Close attention to detail with these steps is important to securing that job of your dreams. Also, keep in mind that while the interview is vital to the prospective employer as they look for the right person for their position, it is your opportunity to decide if a position, or employer, is the right fit for you. Just as the employer will screen out candidates who do not meet the organization's expectations or needs, you should screen out employers who do not fit your expectations and needs.

# CHAPTER 29

# Advice for Choosing a Clinical Fellowship in Audiology and Speech-Language Pathology

Sharon Goodson, MA, CCC-A, NSSLHA President, 2001–2002

## INTRODUCTION

A clinical fellowship (CF) position, sometimes referred to as the clinical fellowship year, is an opportunity for students to practice years of training under the supervision of an ASHA-certified professional. The term CF is also used as a noun to describe a person completing a CF, because during this period you will refer to yourself as a "clinical fellow" to your peers and clients. The CF is the first time you will truly practice most of what you have spent years learning. You will also broaden your professional interests. You will flourish as a clinician if you are in a setting where you feel comfortable and feel like you are contributing to the good of your clients, as well as the clinic. This chapter provides advice for graduate students who are preparing for a CF in audiology or speech-language pathology, and Figure 29-1 is a checklist to track your progress. In addition, Figure 29-2 contains an interview with a CF, providing a glimpse into life in a clinical fellowship.

☐ Consider carefully what you are looking for in a work site.

☐ Start sending out resumés the semester before you graduate.

☐ Talk to professors in your department.

☐ Bring your portfolio with you to interviews.

☐ Ask questions during the interview.

☐ Figure out what qualities and work style you want most in a supervisor.

☐ Consider the differences between types of settings.

**Figure 29-1** Checklist for choosing a clinical fellowship

**An Interview with Sybil Forsythe, CF, CCC-SLP, By Jeremy Saylor, NSSLHA member, University of Kentucky**

As aspiring audiologists and speech-language pathologists, most of us know that in order to apply for your Certificate of Clinical Competence (CCC) from ASHA, you must complete a Clinical Fellowship (CF). I recently sat down with Sybil Forsythe a speech-language pathologist currently fulfilling her CF requirements at a hospital to give an in-depth look at the life of a clinical fellow.

**Q. *Sybil, what was the first day as a CF like?***

**A.** It was very challenging, but familiar. I completed my rotations as a graduate student at the same hospital, which made it convenient because I was already familiar with the staff and how the hospital functioned.

**Q. *What is your CF supervisor like?***

**A.** I am under the supervision of an ASHA-certified SLP who has provided me with excellent guidance and encourages a hands-on approach to therapy.

**Q. *How did you get this position?***

**A.** When I interviewed for this position, I brought along a portfolio that contained a resumé, listed rotations, honors, and scholarships I received. I also included a sample of a newsletter that I had written and edited, as well as a copy of my research thesis, and samples of evaluation reports that I have written.

**Q. *What helped you most during the interview process?***

**A.** I felt very comfortable during the interview because of my previous rotation at the hospital. That also helped me with my salary negotiations. I was able to negotiate my salary and benefits because having worked here, I knew what skill level this hospital needed. I knew that I would be a good asset to the team.

**Q. *What is the age range of the clients that you work with, and what type of disorders are you treating?***

**A.** I work with clients of all ages, from birth to elderly. Most of the clients are ventilator-dependent patients in the Respiratory Care Center. I also have some outpatients that have articulation disorders, language disorders, aphasia, and dysphagia. I like the variety of the patients' ages, disorders, and syndromes.

*(continues)*

**Figure 29-2** Life as a clinical fellow

**Q. *What is the hardest part about your CF?***

**A.** One of the hardest things about my job is when one of my patients has a decline in medical status and/or passes away. Many patients at the Respiratory Care Center are medically fragile. Sometimes babies who are ventilator dependent become very ill. It's hard because your clients are depending on you and can die.

**Q. *What advice do you have for future graduates?***

**A.** I would advise graduates to explore different opportunities and settings and not to jump at the first job offer if it's not exactly what you are seeking. Before you accept your first position, make sure you fully understand the salary, benefits, and what type of caseload you will be working with. Also, find out if the facility offers continuing education and if so, what kind. Last but not least, I would advise students to hang on to your textbooks and notes. They will become a valuable resource that can aid in therapy and research.

**Figure 29-2** (Continued)

# GUIDELINES FOR CHOOSING A CLINICAL FELLOWSHIP IN AUDIOLOGY AND SPEECH-LANGUAGE PATHOLOGY

## Consider Carefully What You Are Looking for in a Work Site

As you work in different settings during your internships and externships, consider what you do and do not like about each setting. Think about both what you can offer a site and what the site can offer you in terms of experiences. Talk to your supervisor about potential openings in the future. It is never too soon to consider your options.

## Start Sending Out Resumés the Semester Before You Graduate

Send resumés to sites that have listed an opening, as well as sites that may not be hiring at this time. Many professional publications, such as *The ASHA Leader*, as well as many career specific Web sites, such as ASHA's Career Center at http://www.audiologyonline.org and http://www.advanceforspanda.com, advertise CF job openings. Realize that it may take six months to a year to find a job, depending on what cities you are searching. Be open to participating in a CF outside of the area where you live or go to school. Sometimes the opportunities are in areas that will require you to relocate.

## Talk to Professors in Your Department

Professors in your department often have close friends and colleagues across the country who may know of clinical fellowship openings. Sometimes, employers send job postings to departments and your professors may have knowledge of these job openings or prospective employers. Your NSSLHA chapter may have a job binder that stores these postings. Use all the resources at hand to help secure a job once you graduate. The professors and resources in your department can be invaluable both now and down the road, if you maintain contact.

## Bring Your Portfolio with You to Interviews

It is especially important to bring any writing samples (e.g., research papers) to interviews. This will give a potential employer a better idea of your capabilities. It also helps them see that you are prepared for the interview.

## Ask Questions During the Interview

The interview is not only a time for the employer to determine if you are a qualified candidate, but it is also your opportunity to determine whether the position, employer, and setting are right for you. When you meet with a potential supervisor, feel free to ask questions in addition to answering questions. You are trying to find a good fit for both you and the employer. Do not be afraid to ask for what you want. When applying for a clinical fellowship, consider asking your potential supervisor the following questions during the interview:

- What types of services are provided to clients?
- Are there any best practice rules or protocols in place?
- How much time will you have to offer?
- Have you supervised a CF before?
- Are they familiar with the requirements of a CF?
- If you have not supervised a CF before, have you worked with students at any level?
- Do clinicians have administrative time set aside, or are their schedules packed with clinic responsibilities?
- Are your audiologists and/or speech-language pathologists ASHA certified?

- Are there any state licensure and/or certification requirements?

- Are you located solely at one site or do you manage many sites?

- Do you have rotating CF positions, or do you expect CFs to work for this facility after the CF is complete? (Some sites have rotating CF positions. When that year is up, the CF moves on. Other sites will not want to invest the time to hire, train, and supervise a CF without the probability that the CF will stay on after ASHA certification.)

- What benefits are there? (Some recommend that you ask this question once you are offered a job.)

- What is the average salary? (Some recommend waiting to negotiate the salary after you are offered a job.)

- Is there a salary increase once certified or fully licensed? (Discuss, up front, what possibility there is for advancement. It is better to learn about these details early. Keep in mind that it can be difficult or impossible to negotiate salary increases once you are in a position; however, again, some recommend asking this question after being offered a job.)

## Figure Out What Qualities and Work Style You Want Most in a Supervisor

While you may not be working closely with your supervisor at all times, you do need to have a good relationship. Make sure that your supervisor is going to be someone who can further your professional interests. Consider whether the supervisor will meet your needs by asking about his or her work style, expectations of employees, and the characteristics he or she values most in an employee. The most important thing is to make sure your supervisor is ASHA certified. The time spent in your CF position will be wasted if your CF supervisor is not ASHA certified. Call the Action Center at 800-498-2071 to verify your supervisor's certification.

## Consider the Differences Between Types of Settings

A larger clinic or hospital will generally offer a broader range of experiences and more interesting cases, but you may encounter more bureaucratic issues, or they may be required to hire fully-licensed clinicians. A smaller clinic or private practice may be easier to work with, but might not offer the variety of experiences a new clinician would benefit from. Take your time to figure out what things matter most to you. This is the first step in your professional future; you do not get a chance to do it over. If you still cannot make up your mind, ask yourself the following questions after each interview:

- Was it clear what would be expected of me? Did this facility do a good job of helping me understand what my caseload would be and the level of responsibility I would have? If the answer is not obvious, it might be a sign that the facility is not organized or that the work environment is tenuous.

- Does this facility care about compensating its employees? What type of employee benefits will this position provide? How flexible is this work environment? Even if they cannot give me the money that I am asking for, is the facility willing to negotiate additional incentives to show that I am valued?

- Did my potential supervisor seem approachable and reasonable? (You will need a supervisor that can answer your questions and explain things clearly. Not everyone is an effective teacher/mentor in an applied setting like a clinic, hospital, or school. Consider how your potential supervisor responds to your questions.) Did he or she give me the information I needed? Does this person seem like someone who is good with conflict resolution? (You are likely to encounter at least some challenges.)

- Will I be working with multiple clinicians with diverse backgrounds? (It is invaluable to work with multiple clinicians and gain from their points of view.)

- Do I see myself working here after my CF is complete? If it is a rotating CF position, would I feel comfortable changing jobs at the end?

- What do I like the most about this CF position? What do I like the least?

- Would I work here for free? (Your reply to this question will really gauge if this is the right position for you. If you would seriously consider working in that setting free of charge, then imagine how great it will be to get a paycheck.)

## CONCLUSION

After many years of education and training, you are finally stepping into a professional role to provide services to individuals with communication disorders. This is the start of what will likely be a long, successful, and enjoyable career. To get off to the right start in your CF, do your homework to determine what setting and employer is the right fit for you. Just as you did when you were applying to undergraduate and graduate programs, research your options and ask questions so that when the time comes to accept a position, you are positive that it is a job in which you will flourish.

# CHAPTER 30

# Going to the ASHA Convention

Marie Patton, NSSLHA President, 2001–2003

## INTRODUCTION

The ASHA Convention is an inspiring experience that all CSD students should attend at least once. Over 10,000 students; audiologists; SLPs; and speech, language, and hearing scientists, parents, and related professionals attend the annual convention each November. When you walk into the spacious convention building, you will probably feel a bit overwhelmed. At the 2003 convention in Chicago, it took 15 to 20 minutes to walk from one end of the convention center to the other. There is so much to see and do that you might miss out if you do not know what to look for. If you have never been to a convention, you probably have questions about what it is like. Read on to find out how to make it a great experience!

## BEFORE THE CONVENTION

### Volunteer at the ASHA Convention

ASHA and NSSLHA will refund the cost of the early bird registration fee to students who are selected to volunteer during the convention. To be chosen as a volunteer, fill out a volunteer application form in May or June. Make sure you have renewed your membership in NSSLHA, since preferences are given to its members.

### Ask If Your NSSLHA Chapter Is Organizing Fundraising Activities for the ASHA Convention

Often, local NSSLHA chapters hold fundraisers to help cover the costs of attending the ASHA Convention. If yours does not, ask if you can set up fundraising activities, such as bake sales or selling candy bars, candles, or cookbooks. Also, some campuses have funds set aside for students to attend educational events. As you might imagine, these funds are not usually advertised. Contact your campus' student organization board to see if you and/or your NSSLHA chapter qualify.

# Register in September to Receive the "Early Bird" Registration Fee

The cost of convention varies from year to year, but members of NSSLHA receive a significant discount. Traditionally, the convention is the week before Thanksgiving, from Thursday until Saturday. However, some years, it is two or three weeks before Thanksgiving. This can be a hectic time for many students, and depending on what your travel plans may be for Thanksgiving, if you want to attend ASHA as well, you should start planning well in advance. The ASHA Web site has information on the cost, location, and dates of the convention each year.

## Register for the Fun NSSLHA Night Activity

While registering for the convention, make sure to sign up for NSSLHA Night, when students and professionals network while having fun, such as a karaoke night, comedy club, or scavenger hunt. Check the NSSLHA Web site in the summer to find out what the NSSLHA Night activity is. Make sure you sign up early; tickets have run out in the first month of registration.

## Register for an ASHA Social Event

ASHA usually hosts something similar to a NSSLHA Night. Most of the attendees will be professionals, but students are more than welcome to attend. In the past, events have been related to shopping and dinner. This can be a fun time, and you will have the opportunity to meet and talk with professionals and students working in a wide range of settings and specialties.

## Find a Place to Stay

If you do not have any friends or relatives to stay with near the convention city, make reservations at a hotel or student hostel. Most students find roommates from their university program and split the cost of a hotel room. ASHA has lists of hotels in the convention city on their Web site. These hotels may have a reduced rate for ASHA Convention attendees and have shuttles to and from the convention center. Some students stay at student hostels, which are found in most major cities. Hostels are places designated specifically for students, where they can stay for a relatively inexpensive rate. They do not come with the amenities of the average hotel, but the prices are much lower. Check the ASHA Web site to identify the student hostel in the city of the next ASHA Convention.

# Make Travel Arrangements for the Convention

Unless you are fortunate enough to live in the convention city, most students fly or drive to the convention. If you look early enough, you might be able to find an affordable flight. Try travel search engines such as http://www.expedia.com and http://www.travelocity.com. However, driving may be cheaper if you can carpool with others and split the cost of gas and parking. Do a search at http://www.mapquest.com to see how far the convention is from your front door. If you opt to drive, call your hotel to see if you have to pay extra for parking.

# Plan Your Commute to the Convention Center from Where You Stay

While there may be AHSA-provided shuttles to and from some hotels, it may not be available where you are staying. Therefore, expect to take public transportation, such as a bus, train, or subway. Walking is always an option if you are within a few miles of the convention center. Your hotel or the hostel can assist you in finding the best way to get to the convention center.

# Select the Courses You Want to Attend

On the ASHA Convention Web page, you can view and/or download the convention program book and create a schedule of all courses you want to attend. The schedule includes times, dates, and room numbers. The site allows you to read through abstracts to identify what interests you the most. The following are some of the educational events you can attend.

***Poster Presentations.*** In poster presentations, investigators summarize their research on a poster and give you a brief explanation. Many poster presentations are given in a gigantic room. Attendees can walk up and down the rows of posters and stop to read the posters that interest them. Usually someone from the research team is present to explain the poster. Presentations change throughout the day, so it is helpful to identify when the posters that interest you will be available by looking on the ASHA Web site.

***ASHA Sessions.*** During the ASHA sessions, speakers usually discuss their cutting-edge research. Some sessions are at the introductory level and others are at the advanced level. If a topic interests you or corresponds to a research project you are working on, be sure to arrive early to get a good seat.

***NSSLHA Sessions.*** Traditionally, NSSLHA has some sessions that are specifically geared toward students. Sessions in the past have been about the Praxis examination, clinical fellowships, job settings, and resumés. Sometimes, NSSLHA hosts sessions about topics specifically related to the field, such as "Everything You Need to Know about Auditory Processing." Find out what sessions are being offered at the convention you are planning to attend and sign up to attend. Again, arrive early to get a good seat.

***Workshops.*** An ASHA Special Interest Division usually sponsors workshops the day or two before the convention begins. Speakers usually give extensive talks about a disorder and how to treat it. However, the topics can vary. You usually need to pre-register for workshops and pay extra. If you are a member of the ASHA Special Interest Division that hosts it, you can usually receive a significant discount. Refer to Chapter 32 for more information about Special Interest Divisions.

## Bring Your Nametag and Convention Registration Materials to the Convention

ASHA will mail you a nametag and tickets for any pre-registered events (e.g., NSSLHA Night Activity). Make sure to bring these along with you to the convention. Do not forget to pack your list of sessions you want to attend.

## Bring a Good Pair of Walking Shoes, Professional Clothing, and Business Cards

If you have never attended a convention or event at a major convention center before, you will most likely be amazed at how huge these buildings are. Once you are in the convention center, you will be doing a lot of walking between sessions, events, and the exhibitor hall where products and services are featured. Plus, you will most likely be walking to and from your hotel or to other points of interest in the city. Good walking shoes are a must! You will be interacting with many professionals, some of whom are highly respected and influential in the field, and you will want to present yourself as a professional as well. You should wear professional clothing that is comfortable (e.g., women can wear dress pants and a blouse or business skirt set; men can wear dress pants, shirt, and tie and dress jacket if preferred). While jeans and casual clothing are not prohibited, this is a professional event, and you should show respect to your colleagues by dressing appropriately. Also bring business cards, which are helpful because you will do a lot of networking. You will interact with professionals and students who you may want to keep in contact with after the convention. If you or a friend has a computer and printer, you can easily purchase business card paper from an office supply store and use a word processing program (e.g., Microsoft Word) to format your own cards.

## Bring Extra Money

Accidents and unexpected events can happen. If you are driving, your car could break down and you will need to pay for repairs. If you are flying, your flight might be delayed or canceled, and you may need to buy food. Be prepared so you are not stranded anywhere.

## Save Money by Bringing Some of Your Own Snacks or Attend Convention Events That Offer Food

Buying snacks at the convention center or airport will be costly. Bring non-perishable food and beverages, such as granola bars, fruits, chips, and water. If your hotel or hostel has a refrigerator and microwave, bring sandwiches and frozen meals so you do not have to go to a restaurant for breakfast, lunch, and dinner. Often, events are planned that provide food. Plan to attend those events and make sure you eat.

# DURING THE CONVENTION

## Attend the First-Timers Breakfast

ASHA hosts a breakfast for all attendees (including students) who have never been to an ASHA Convention. This is a great way to meet other first-timers. The breakfast is usually held on Thursday morning.

## Attend the Graduate School Fair (GSF) If You Are Applying to a Doctoral or Master's Program

The Graduate School Fair is an opportunity for students to meet with representatives from graduate programs to learn more about doctoral- and master's-level CSD programs, and to get information about funding opportunities. Attending the Graduate School Fair is an easy way to learn about programs that you are interested in attending, without having to travel to each location.

## Attend the ASHA Placement Center/Job Fair If You Are Graduating in the Next Year

You can speak with potential employers throughout the country to search for a clinical fellowship (CF). Bring a copy of your resumé and wear professional clothing because you will go through interviews on the spot. Make sure you get the business cards of those places that interest you the most. Call the company/employer within a week or two after the convention to express that you are interested in the position.

## Attend the Key Note Speaker Presentation

Usually, ASHA arranges for a motivating and insightful speaker to kick-off the convention. Make sure to attend this event, as it is often memorable and inspiring.

## Attend the Honors Ceremony

The Honors Ceremony is an exciting event where thousands of attendees celebrate the accomplishments of ASHA members. It is like the Academy Awards for audiologists, hearing scientists, speech-language pathologists, and speech-language scientists. Movie clips are played that star those who have earned the highest honors of the Associations: ASHA Honors. NSSLHA also presents its Editorial Award and NSSLHA Honors during the ASHA Awards Ceremony.

## Attend the Exhibit Hall

The giant exhibit hall is filled with companies and services displaying and selling their most up-to-date products. You will find publishers selling books and software, usually at a significant discount. In fact, if you know that you need a particular book for an upcoming class, you may want to take advantage of the special convention discount. You can also pick up a lot of freebies at this event, such as tote bags, pens, highlighters, key chains, penlights (that are especially good for oral mechanism exams), and notepads. However, choose wisely when taking items. Otherwise, you can end up with a lot of unnecessary junk to pack and bring back with you on the plane. The exhibit hall is usually open on Thursday, Friday, and Saturday of convention.

## Attend the NSSLHA Executive Council Meeting

The NSSLHA Executive Council meeting is open to conference attendees. The place and time of the meetings are listed on the *ASHA Convention Daily Newspaper* and NSSLHA convention brochure located throughout the convention center.

## Visit the NSSLHA Booth

When visiting the exhibit hall, be sure to stop by the NSSLHA booth. NSSLHA usually gives away neat gifts to students (one year, they gave away CD cases). You can pick up the NSSLHA convention brochure and ask any questions about the convention, NSSLHA membership, or academic issues. The booth is usually in the exhibit hall.

## Visit the ASHA Service Center

Spend some time at the ASHA service center. ASHA also gives away some nice gifts (e.g., lighted keychains, tote bags) and has useful information related to ASHA certification, membership, Special Interest Divisions, journals, and resources available exclusively to ASHA and NSSLHA members.

## CONCLUSION

The ASHA Convention has much to offer students and professionals in CSD. You can learn about the most cutting-edge research, attend sessions pertaining to your particular areas of interest, access a wide range of products and services in the exhibit hall, find out more about potential graduate schools and job opportunities, and of course, meet CSD students from around the country for some fun social events. It is everything related to speech, language, hearing, and swallowing, all in one place, at one time. Attending the convention as a student is excellent preparation for attending it later as a certified practicing professional.

# CHAPTER 31

# ASHA Certification

Georgia McMann, Director of Certification Administration, ASHA

## INTRODUCTION

Once you have received your graduate degree you will want to apply for ASHA certification in either audiology or speech-language pathology. This chapter covers the current certification standards for SLPs and audiologists, as well as the new certification standards effective January 1, 2006 for SLPs newly applying for certification and January 1, 2008 for audiologists newly applying for certification. This chapter provides an overview of these requirements. For more detailed information, visit the ASHA Web site or contact ASHA directly.

## CURRENT CERTIFICATION STANDARDS

The current certification standards went into effect in 1993. For both audiology and SLP, the standards mandate that applicants for certification have a graduate degree, either a master's or a doctorate. Current standards also require that all applicants complete a supervised post-graduate experience, called a clinical fellowship (CF), and that all applicants successfully complete the Praxis examination in their area of desired certification.

For individuals applying for certification in audiology, there must be at least 75 semester hours of coursework overall, with the following breakdown:

- 27 semester hours of coursework in the basic sciences, to include:
  - 6 semester hours in biological/physical sciences and mathematics
  - 6 semester hours in behavioral and/or social sciences
  - 15 semester hours in basic human communication processes; this must include at least one course in anatomic and physiologic bases, one course in physical and psychophysical bases, and one course in linguistic and psycholinguistic aspects
- 36 semester hours of coursework in the professional area of audiology, 30 of which must be at the graduate level, with at least 21 semester hours completed at the graduate level in audiology. At least 6 semester hours must be completed in auditory pathology and 6 semester hours

must be in habilitative/rehabilitative audiology. Additionally, there must be at least 6 semester hours of coursework in speech and language pathology, 3 semester hours in speech, and 3 semester hours in language.

Practicum requirements under current standards require the following:

- 25 clock hours of clinical observation prior to beginning initial clinical practicum
- 350 total clock hours of supervised clinical practicum, 250 of which must be at the graduate level in audiology
- 20 clock hours of clinical practicum in speech-language pathology unrelated to hearing impairments
- Of the 250 clock hours in audiology, there must be a distribution of:
  - 40 clock hours in evaluation of hearing with children
  - 40 clock hours of evaluation of hearing with adults
  - 40 clock hours of selection and use of amplification and assistive devices for children
  - 40 clock hours of selection and use of amplification and assistive devices for adults
  - 20 clock hours of treatment of hearing disorders in children and adults

Individuals applying for certification in speech-language pathology must present at least 75 semester hours of coursework overall, with the following break-down:

- 27 semester hours of coursework in the basic sciences, to include:
  - 6 semester hours in biological/physical sciences and mathematics
  - 6 semester hours in behavioral and/or social sciences
  - 15 semester hours in basic human communication processes; this must include at least one course in anatomic and physiologic bases, one course in physical and psychophysical bases, and one course in linguistic and psycholinguistic aspects
- 36 semester hours of coursework in the professional area of speech-language pathology, 30 of which must be at the graduate level, with at least 21 semester hours completed at the graduate level in speech. At least 6 semester hours must be completed in speech disorders and 6 semester hours must be in language disorders. Additionally, there must be at least 6 semester hours of coursework in audiology, 3 semester hours in hearing disorders and hearing evaluation, and 3 semester hours in habilitative/rehabilitative procedures.

Practicum requirements under current speech standards require the following:

- 25 clock hours of clinical observation prior to beginning initial clinical practicum

- 350 clock hours total of clinical practicum, with at least 250 clock hours at the graduate level in speech-language pathology

- 20 clock hours of practicum in audiology

- Of the 250 clock hours required in speech, they must be distributed as follows:

  - 20 clock hours of evaluation of speech disorders with children
  - 20 clock hours of evaluation of speech disorders with adults
  - 20 clock hours of evaluation of language disorders with children
  - 20 clock hours of evaluation of language disorders with adults
  - 20 clock hours of treatment of speech disorders with children
  - 20 clock hours of treatment of speech disorders with adults
  - 20 clock hours of treatment of language disorders with children
  - 20 clock hours of treatment of language disorders with adults

Individuals will have until December 31, 2005 to apply for certification under the current speech-language pathology standards and until December 31, 2007 to apply under the current audiology standards. After those dates, applicants will be required to apply for certification under the new standards. For more information on current certification standards, visit the ASHA Web site at http://www.asha.org and search for certification standards.

## NEW CERTIFICATION STANDARDS IN AUDIOLOGY

New audiology standards will go into effect in two phases. The first phase, effective January 1, 2007, requires that applicants complete 75 semester hours of post-baccalaureate education culminating in a doctoral or other recognized graduate degree, and includes academic coursework and a minimum of 12 months of full-time equivalent, supervised clinical practicum. The course of study must address the knowledge and skills pertinent to the field of audiology.

The new audiology standards require that applicants have a foundation of prerequisite knowledge and skills, including:

- skills in oral and written or other forms of communication
- skills and knowledge of life sciences, physical sciences, behavioral sciences, and mathematics, demonstrated through transcript credit for a course in each of the four areas

Additionally, applicants for certification in audiology must have acquired knowledge and developed skills in four areas: foundations of practice, prevention and identification, evaluation, and treatment. These new standards require assessment of the student's acquisition of the specified knowledge and skills by the graduate academic program. Clinical practicum must include direct observation, guidance, and feedback by the supervisor to permit the student to monitor, evaluate, and improve performance and to develop clinical competence. Supervisors of practicum that will be used for ASHA certification must hold current ASHA certification. Under these new audiology standards, there will be no CF; however, applicants for certification will still be required to successfully complete the Praxis examination in audiology.

The second phase of the audiology standards will become effective January 1, 2012. After this date, all applicants for certification will be required to have an earned doctoral degree. For ASHA certification purposes, the degree can be a Ph.D., an Ed.D., a Sc.D., or the AuD.

More information on the new audiology standards is located on the ASHA Web site at http://www.asha.org under the audiology certification standards.

## NEW CERTIFICATION STANDARDS
## IN SPEECH-LANGUAGE PATHOLOGY

The new speech-language pathology certification standards become effective January 1, 2005. These standards mandate 75 semester hours of coursework overall, including at least 36 semester hours at the graduate level. The program of study must address the knowledge and skills pertinent to the field of speech-language pathology. Further, the new standards require that the applicant have transcript credit in each of the following areas:

- biological science
- physical science
- mathematics
- the social/behavioral sciences

Applicants, under new 2005 standards, must demonstrate knowledge of basic human communication and swallowing processes, including their biological, neurological, acoustic, psychological, developmental, and linguistic and cultural bases. Also, the applicant must demonstrate knowledge of the nature of speech, language, hearing, and communication disorders and differences, and swallowing disorders, including the etiologies, characteristics, anatomical/physiological, acoustic, psychological, developmental, and linguistic and cultural correlates in nine areas. Additionally, applicants must demonstrate knowledge of standards of ethical conduct, processes used in research and the integration of research principles into evidence-based clinical practice, contemporary professional issues, and knowledge of certification, specialty recognition, licensure, and other relevant professional credentials. As in audiology, applicants for certification in speech will be required to possess skill in oral and written or other forms of communication.

With regard to clinical practicum, applicants will be required to have completed a minimum of 400 clock hours of supervised experience in speech-language pathology. Of those, 25 hours must be spent in clinical observation and 375 hours must be spent in direct client/patient contact. Of the 375 hours of client/patient contact, 325 must be completed while engaged in graduate study, and individuals holding current ASHA certification in speech-language pathology must supervise all hours used for ASHA certification.

After completion of the academic coursework and supervised clinical practicum, applicants must successfully complete a Speech-Language Pathology Clinical Fellowship (SLPCF). This experience must consist of the equivalent of 36 weeks of full-time clinical experience with a mentoring speech-language pathologist who holds current certification in speech-language pathology. And finally, applicants for certification under the new standards will be required to pass the Praxis examination in speech-language pathology.

Detailed information on the new speech-language pathology standards can be found on the ASHA Web site at http://www.asha.org under SLP certification standards.

## CERTIFICATION MAINTENANCE

Individuals holding ASHA certification are required to maintain that certification through annual payment of dues/fees and, beginning January 1, 2003 in audiology and January 1, 2005 in speech, through participation in continuing professional development activities. The renewal period is three years and mandates the accumulation of 30 hours of continuing professional development during each renewal period. This requirement applies to all certificate holders, regardless of the date they originally became certified.

Professional development is defined as any activity that relates to the science and contemporary practice of audiology, speech-language pathology, and speech/language/hearing sciences, and results in the acquisition of new knowledge and skills or the enhancement of current knowledge and skills. Certification maintenance requirements for both audiology and speech and FAQs can be found on the ASHA Web site at http://www.asha.org under certification maintenance.

## CONCLUSION

While the standards for certification are quite detailed, the benefits of certification are many:

- Certification is the public's assurance that an individual has met rigorous, peer-developed and reviewed standards endorsed by a national professional body.
- Employers welcome and respect certification by a national body.
- Certification limits liability claims.
- Certification is a fundamental standard among major health professions in this country.
- Certification is important for internal professional recognition, external verification, and accountability.

For over 75 years, ASHA has been the guardian of the professions of audiology; speech-language pathology; and speech, language, and hearing sciences. Take the time to learn about the ASHA certification program and you will see that it is the symbol of quality that you will desire.

# CHAPTER 32

# Being Active in the American Speech-Language-Hearing Association

Marie Patton, masters's student, SLP, University of Wisconsin-Madison and NSSLHA President, 2001–2003

## INTRODUCTION

Once you make the transition from a student to a professional, you can convert your membership from NSSLHA to ASHA. As an ASHA member, you have the opportunity to further the profession by contributing your experiences and talents by serving on boards, councils, and committees. To learn more about how ASHA is organized, see Figure 32-1, which presents the ASHA governance chart. To get the most out of ASHA membership, learn more about the purpose and mission of these boards, councils, and committees that you can join. Remember that any professional association is only as strong as its members. It is your responsibility to become an active member of the professional association.

## ASHA GOVERNANCE

The Legislative Council (LC) and the Executive Board (EB) are at the head of the Association. Legislative Councilors and EB officers are elected by ASHA members to serve the Association, address problems that members are having, and create focus initiatives (goals of the Association that are usually over a period of years and are financially supported in the budget).

The 150-member Legislative Council consists of two bodies: the Audiology/Hearing Science (A/HS) Assembly and the Speech-Language Pathology/Speech-Language Science (SLP/SLS) Assembly. Assembly members debate and vote on resolutions that specifically relate to A/HS or SLP/SLS. When resolutions address both assemblies (e.g., the budget of the Association), the entire LC debates and votes on the resolutions.

## ASHA BOARDS

Following is a list of ASHA Boards to consider joining. ASHA members must complete a Volunteer Pool Form to be considered for positions on these Boards. A Volunteer Pool Form is available in the ASHA membership application or can be downloaded from the Governance page of the ASHA Web site.

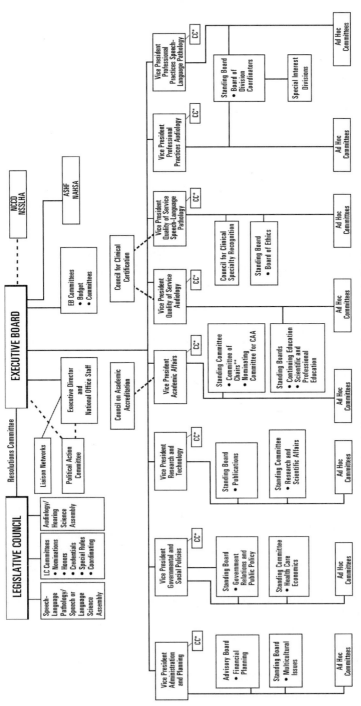

**Figure 32-1** American Speech-Language-Hearing Association governance structure

- Board of Ethics
- Multicultural Issues Board (MIB)
- Continuing Education Board
- Publications Board
- Financial Planning Board (FPB)
- Governmental Relations and Public Policy Board (GRPP)
- Scientific and Professional Education Board (SPEB)
- Special Interest Divisions Board of Division Coordinators (Divisions)

# ASHA COMMITTEES AND COUNCILS

Following is a list of committees and councils that you might consider when you become a member of ASHA. Check with the Executive Office about the requirements to serve on these, as they vary by committee. Detailed information about the purpose and operation of these committees and councils is available on the Governance page of the ASHA Web site located at http://www.asha.org.

- Academic Affairs Coordinating Committee (AACC)
- Administration and Planning Coordinating Committee (APCC)
- The Committee on Budget
- The Committee on Committees
- The Committee on Corporate Relations Planning (CCRP)
- The Committee on Credentials
- The Committee on Honors
- The Committee on Nominations and Elections
- The Committee on Resolutions
- The Committee on Special Rules
- The Council for Clinical Certification in Audiology & Speech-Language Pathology
- Council for Clinical Specialty Recognition
- The Council of Editors
- The Council on Academic Accreditation in Audiology and Speech-Language Pathology
- The Governmental and Social Policies Coordinating Committee
- Health Care Economics Committee
- Joint Committee of the American Speech-Language-Hearing Association and the American Academy of Otolaryngology—Head and Neck Surgery
- Joint Committee of the American Speech-Language-Hearing Association and Council on Education of the Deaf
- Joint Committee for the Communication Needs of Persons with Severe Disabilities
- Joint Committee on Infant Hearing

- Joint Committee on Interprofessional Relationships with Neuropsychology
- Joint Committee on State-National Association Relationships
- Legislative Council Agenda-Setting Group
- Legislative Council Coordinating Committee
- National Joint Committee for the Communication Needs of Persons with Severe Disabilities
- National Joint Committee on Learning Disabilities
- Nominating Committee for the Council on Academic Accreditation
- Political Action Committee (PAC)
- Professional Practices in Audiology Coordinating Committee
- Professional Practices in Speech-Language Pathology Coordinating Committee
- Quality of Service in Audiology Coordinating Committee
- Quality of Service Speech-Language Pathology Coordinating Committee
- Research and Scientific Affairs Committee
- Research and Technology Coordinating Committee
- ASHA Caucuses (groups that usually meet at the ASHA Convention to discuss issues relating to professionals and clients who are of the subsequent cultures): Asian-Indian Caucus (AIC), Asian Pacific Islander Caucus, Hispanic Caucus, Native American Caucus, Lesbian/Gay/ Bisexual Audiologists and Speech-Language Pathologists (L'GASP)

## ASHA SPECIAL INTEREST DIVISIONS

NSSLHA members may become Associate Affiliates of any of the ASHA Special Interest Divisions (Divisions) at a significantly reduced fee. All Divisions have newsletters with articles that can be used to receive continuing education units. Some Divisions hold conferences during the year and/or a workshop during the ASHA Convention that NSSLHA members can attend at a discounted rate. More detailed information about the following Special Interest Division is available on the ASHA Web site at http://www.asha.org:

- Division 1: Language Learning and Education
- Division 2: Neurophysiology and Neurogenic Speech and Language Disorders
- Division 3: Voice and Voice Disorders
- Division 4: Fluency and Fluency Disorders
- Division 5: Speech Science and Orofacial Disorders
- Division 6: Hearing and Hearing Disorders: Research and Diagnostics
- Division 7: Aural Rehabilitation and Its Instrumentation
- Division 8: Hearing Conservation and Occupational Audiology
- Division 9: Hearing and Hearing Disorders in Childhood
- Division 10: Issues in Higher Education
- Division 11: Administration and Supervision

- Division 12: Augmentative and Alternative Communication
- Division 13: Swallowing and Swallowing Disorders (Dysphagia)
- Division 14: Communication Disorders and Sciences in Culturally and Linguistically Diverse (CLD) Populations
- Division 15: Gerontology
- Division 16: School-Based Issues

## WHAT YOU CAN DO TO BE A GOOD PROFESSIONAL

As a professional, you have several options in what you can do to be an active volunteer in associations. The following suggestions can be accomplished throughout your professional career. Some of these are good to do every year (e.g., renew memberships), whereas others would be great if you could do them at least once (e.g., visit a local high school to promote the professions).

- Renew memberships (e.g., state association membership, ASHA certification, and ASHA membership).
- Earn continuing education credits (CEUs) and continue ASHA certification.
- Participate in Better Hearing and Speech Month (BHSM) every May. ASHA usually provides free materials that you can pass out to parents, professionals, and the public.
- Donate to the ASHA Political Action Committee (PAC) and your state association's PAC (if one exists).
- Be a clinical fellowship supervisor if you think that you have good teaching skills.
- Be a site supervisor for graduate students (e.g., for AuD students who are gaining clinical experience off-campus).
- Donate to the American Speech-Language-Hearing Foundation. ASHF is a non-profit organization that supports various causes in CSD and offer scholarships to students.
- Report unethical behavior of fellow ASHA members to the ASHA Board of Ethics. Consult with the board to resolve these issues. Also, contact the board if you are questioning what you are doing as a clinician.
- Be a mentor to students who are interested in the field.
- Attend state and ASHA conventions.
- Attend the ASHA Legislative Council meeting at the ASHA Convention.
- Nominate yourself to be an ASHA Legislative Councilor for your state.
- Nominate yourself to run for an ASHA Executive Board position.
- Nominate yourself to be a NSSLHA Consultant when a position is available, or volunteer to be a NSSLHA Chapter Advisor if you are on faculty at a university. These are great ways to mentor students.

- Volunteer to be on a committee for ASHA. Print out and complete the volunteer form.
- Nominate yourself to be an officer for your state association.
- Contact your ASHA Legislative Councilor when there is a professional problem that should be addressed by ASHA (e.g. reimbursements, specialty certification, shortages of professionals, etc.)
- Remain active in ASHA Special Interest Divisions.
- Participate in Peer Reviews online.
- Sign up for the ASHA Continuing Education registry and allow ASHA to keep track of your CEUs.
- Register the place where you work on Proserv, if it is not already registered. Visit the Consumer channel of the ASHA Web site to register. Proserv is a free service that is provided by ASHA to help consumers find certified audiologists and speech-language pathologists.
- Consider a researcher-clinician partnership to pursue clinical research. ASHA has a number of electronic resources including *ASHA Research Electronic Newsletter, Research Voice: ASHA's Research ListServ,* and *Researcher Referral System.*
- Consider earning your doctoral degree if you do not already have one.
- Apply for specialty recognition through ASHA. Currently, the three areas of specialty recognition are Child Language, Fluency, and Swallowing.
- Consider visiting local high schools and encourage students to become audiologists and SLPs. Contact NSSLHA or ASHA for current recruitment tips and materials.

## CONCLUSION

Being a good audiologist, speech-language pathologist, or speech-language-hearing scientist can mean many things. It can mean providing high quality service to clients; performing careful, meaningful research that furthers the collective understanding of the field; being not only highly educated and specially trained, but continuing to educate yourself throughout the course of your career; and serving as a mentor to new students, clinicians, and researchers. Being a good audiologist, speech-language pathologist, or speech-language-hearing scientist can also mean participating in and giving back to the professional organization that unites, serves, certifies, and supports the profession. This chapter provides a brief glimpse into the many ways—large and small—that you can be involved with ASHA. Although you do not need to do all that is suggested in this chapter, these are at least some ways for you to become more involved in the profession. NSSLHA, ASHA, the field of communication sciences, and the many individuals with communication disorders and their families look forward to the contributions you will make during your career.

## Organizational Tools

You will need to be highly organized to succeed as an undergraduate, graduate student, clinician, researcher, and/or professor. Each year you are in school, your organizational needs are likely to increase. Here are some suggestions to help you learn how to be highly organized.

## PURCHASE ORGANIZATIONAL SCHOOL SUPPLIES

- A 1 1/2- to 2-inch binder for each class (although at the beginning of the semester, you can combine several classes into one binder)
- Sticky labels for binders (or a permanent marker to write on binders)
- 5 to 6 dividers or Post-It® notes for each class:
  - For regular courses, divide into *syllabus, notes, assignments, handouts,* and *study guides.*
  - For clinical courses, divide into *syllabus, notes from lectures, notes from meetings with clinical instructor, to do lists to prepare for client sessions, feedback from clinical instructor,* and *handouts.*
- Loose-leaf paper for binders
- Spiral or bound notebooks or paper for binders to take notes in each class
- Pen/pencil case to carry supplies to classes
- Pens and pencils
- Highlighters
- Whiteout
- Small Post-It® notes
- Tab dispenser
- Paper clips
- Hole puncher (electric or manual)
- Regular stapler with extra staples
- Labels with your name and email address for all of your textbooks, binders, and planner (you never know when you might lose them)
- Business card paper to create your own business cards

- Phone card (to use to call professors and classmates if you do not have a cell phone or are out of minutes)
- Large weekly and monthly planner
- Thank you cards

## PURCHASE USEFUL ELECTRONIC DEVICES AND TOOLS

- Floppy disks
- Blank CDs (if you have access to a CD writer)
- USB Flash Drive (remember to back up your files often)
- Personal Digital Assistant (PDA) or a large weekly and monthly planner (depending on if you would like and can afford a PDA); many PDAs come with expandable keyboards that you can use to type your notes during class or a meeting
- Personal computer (desktop or laptop) with a word processing program, such as Microsoft® Word
- Printer (if you can afford it, purchase one with a fax and copier; there are some affordable models available if you look for them)
- Extra print cartridges
- Extra computer paper
- Internet access (some universities have free Internet access for students)
- Otoscope
- Digital recorder (e.g., for language samples)
- Calculator

## PURCHASE USEFUL FURNITURE

- Desk
- Comfortable desk chair
- Printer cart (if your desk does not have space for a printer)
- Bookcases (for all of your binders and textbooks)
- Bright desk lamp

# APPENDIX B

## Undergraduate and Graduate Programs in CSD

**KEY TO PROGRAM OFFERINGS**

| | | |
|---|---|---|
| i | = | Accredited by the CAA |
| ii | = | Not Accredited by the CAA |
| iii | = | Undergraduate Program |
| iv | = | Audiology master's program |
| v | = | SLP masters program |
| vi | = | Doctor of Audiology program |
| vii | = | Doctor of Philosophy program (clinical track available) |
| viii | = | Doctor of Science program |
| ix | = | Doctor of Speech-Language and Audiology |
| x | = | Bi-lingual/Minority Emphasis Program |
| xi | = | Historically Black College or University |
| xii | = | Distance Learning Program |

### ALABAMA

ALABAMA A&M UNIVERSITY
Department of Special Education
(256) 851-5533
http://www.aamu.edu
Program Offerings: **i, iii, v, xi**

AUBURN UNIVERSITY
Department of Communication Disorders
(334) 844-9600
http://www.auburn.edu
Program Offerings: **i, iv, v, vi**

AUBURN UNIVERSITY – MONTGOMERY
Department of Communication and Dramatic
   Arts
(334) 244-3379
http://www.aum.edu/home/academics/
   schools/libarts/dept/cdarts/cdarts/
   commdram.htm
Program Offerings: **ii, iii**

UNIVERSITY OF ALABAMA
Department of Communicative Disorders
(205) 348-7131
http://www.as.ua.edu/comdis/
Program Offerings: **i, v, iii**

UNIVERSITY OF MONTEVALLO
Department of Communication Science &
   Disorders
(205) 665-6720
http://www.montevallo.edu/csd/
   Gradslp.shtm
Program Offerings: **i, iii, v**

UNIVERSITY OF SOUTH ALABAMA
Department of Speech Pathology & Audiology
(251) 380-2600
http://www.southalabama.edu/
   speechandhearing
Program Offerings: **i, iii, iv, v, vi, vii**

### ARIZONA

ARIZONA SCHOOL OF HEALTH SCIENCES
Department of Audiology
(480) 219-6020
http://www.ashs.edu
Program Offerings: **i, vi**

ARIZONA STATE UNIVERSITY
Department of Speech & Hearing Science
(480) 965-2374
http://www.asu.edu/clas/shs
Program Offerings: **i, iii, iv, v, vi, vii, x**

NORTHERN ARIZONA UNIVERSITY
Department of Communication Sciences &
   Disorders
(928) 523-2969
http://www.nau.edu
Program Offerings: **i, iii, v**

UNIVERSITY OF ARIZONA
Department of Speech & Hearing Sciences
(520) 621-1644
http://w3.arizona.edu/~sphweb/
Program Offerings: **i, iii, iv, v, vii, x**

## ARKANSAS

ARKANSAS STATE UNIVERSITY
Program in Communication Disorders
(870) 972-3106
http://www.graduateschool.astate.edu/
   spcomth.htm
Program Offerings: **i, iii, v**

HARDING UNIVERSITY
Communication Disorders Program
(501) 279-4445
http://www.harding.edu/CD/index.html
Program Offerings: **ii, iii**

OUACHITA BAPTIST UNIVERSITY
Department of Speech Communication
(870) 245-5000
http://www.obu.edu/speech/
Program Offerings: **ii, iii**

UNIVERSITY OF ARKANSAS, FAYETTEVILLE
Department of Rehabilitation, Human
   Resources, and Communication Disorders
(479) 575-4509
http://www.uark.edu/Departments/coehp/
   CDIS.htm
Program Offerings: **i, v**

UNIVERSITY OF ARKANSAS, LITTLE ROCK
Department of Audiology & Speech Pathology
(501) 569-3155
http://www.uams.edu/chrp/audiospeech/
   default.asp
Program Offerings: **i, iii, iv, v**

UNIVERSITY OF CENTRAL ARKANSAS
Department of Speech-Language Pathology
(501) 450-3176
http://faculty.uca.edu/~sharonr/degree.htm
Program Offerings: **i, iii, v**

## CALIFORNIA

BIOLA UNIVERSITY
School of Arts and Sciences
(562) 903-6000
http://www.biola.edu/sas/
Program Offerings: **ii, iii**

CALIFORNIA STATE UNIVERSITY, CHICO
Department of Communication Arts &
   Sciences/SPPA Program
(530) 898-4379
http://www.csuchico.edu/gisp/gs/programs/
   cmsd/index.html
Program Offerings: **i, iii, v**

CALIFORNIA STATE UNIVERSITY, FRESNO
Department of Communicative Sciences &
   Disorders
(559) 278-2423
http://www.csufresno.edu/gradstudies/
   narratives/disorder-prog.htm
Program Offerings: **i, iii, v**

CALIFORNIA STATE UNIVERSITY, FULLERTON
Speech Communication/Communicative
   Disorders Program
(714) 278-3617
http://www.communications.fullerton.edu
Program Offerings: **i, iii, v**

CALIFORNIA STATE UNIVERSITY, HAYWARD
Department of Communicative Sciences &
   Disorders
(510) 885-3233
http://www.csuhayward.edu/ecat/20022003/
   u-sppa.html#section10
Program Offerings: **i, iii, v**

CALIFORNIA STATE UNIVERSITY,
   LONG BEACH
Department of Communicative Disorders
(562) 985-4594
http://www.csulb.edu/Departments/
   comm-disorders
Program Offerings: **ii, iii, iv, v, x**

CALIFORNIA STATE UNIVERSITY,
   LOS ANGELES
Department of Communication Disorders
(323) 343-4754
http://www.calstatela.edu/Department/com_
   dis/index.htm
Program Offerings: **i, iii, iv, v**

CALIFORNIA STATE UNIVERSITY,
NORTHRIDGE
Department of Communication Disorders &
Sciences
(818) 677-2852
http://hhd.csun.edu/comdis/
Program Offerings: **i, iii, iv, v**

CALIFORNIA STATE UNIVERSITY,
SACRAMENTO
Department of Speech Pathology & Audiology
(916) 278-7341
http://www.hhs.csus.edu/SPA/
Program Offerings: **i, iii, iv, v**

LOMA LINDA UNIVERSITY
Department of Speech-Language
Pathology/Audiology
(909) 558-4998
http://www.llu.edu/llu/sahp/speech/
Program Offerings: **i, iii, v**

SAN DIEGO STATE UNIVERSITY
School of Speech, Language, and Hearing
Sciences
(619) 594-7746
http://arweb.sdsu.edu/es/psc/ab/
commdisorders.htm
Program Offerings: **i, iii, iv, v, vi, vii, x**

SAN DIEGO STATE UNIVERSITY
Au.D. Joint Doctoral Program (SDSU/UCSD)
School of Speech, Language, Hearing
Sciences
(619) 594-6140
http://chhs.sdsu.edu/slhs/
Program Offerings: **i, vi**

SAN FRANCISCO STATE UNIVERSITY
Department of Special Education,
Communicative Disorders Program
(415) 338-1001
http://www.sfsu.edu/~bulletin/current/
programs/speech.htm#544
Program Offerings: **i, iii, iv, v**

SAN JOSE STATE UNIVERSITY
Communication Disorders & Sciences
Program
(408) 924-3688
http://info.sjsu.edu/web-dbgen/catalog/
departments/COMM-section-5.html
Program Offerings: **i, iii, v**

UNIVERSITY OF CALIFORNIA –
SANTA BARBARA
Department of Speech and Hearing Sciences
(805) 893-2684
http://www.catalog.ucsb.edu/LS/speech.htm
Program Offerings: **ii, iii**

UNIVERSITY OF REDLANDS
Department of Communicative Disorders
(909) 335-4061
http://www.redlands.edu
Program Offerings: **i, iii, v**

UNIVERSITY OF THE PACIFIC
Department of Speech-Language Pathology
(209) 946-3233
http://www.pacific.edu/homepage/
graduate/SPLP.asp
Program Offerings: **i, iii, v**

## CANADA

MCGILL UNIVERSITY
School of Communication Sciences and
Disorders
(514) 398-4137
http://www.mcgill.ca/scsd
Program Offerings: **i, v, vii**

UNIVERSITY OF TORONTO
Graduate Department of Speech-Language
Pathology
(416) 978-2770
http://www.slp.utoronto.ca
Program Offerings: **i, v, vii**

## COLORADO

METROPOLITAN STATE COLLEGE OF DENVER
School of Letter, Arts and Sciences
(303) 556-3033
http://www.mscd.edu/academic/scolas/spe/
spefacts.html
Program Offerings: **ii, iii**

UNIVERSITY OF COLORADO AT BOULDER
Department of Speech-Language & Hearing
Sciences
(303) 492-5284
http://www.colorado.edu
Program Offerings: **i, iii, iv, v, vi, vii**

UNIVERSITY OF NORTHERN COLORADO
Department of Communication Disorders
(970) 351-2734
http://www.unco.edu
Program Offerings: **i, iii, iv, v, vi**

## CONNECTICUT

SOUTHERN CONNECTICUT STATE
   UNIVERSITY
Department of Communication Disorders
(203) 392-5954
http://www.southernct.edu/departments/
   graduatestudies/gpofferingsCmd.php3
Program Offerings: **i, iii, iv, v**

UNIVERSITY OF CONNECTICUT
Department of Communication Sciences
(860) 486-2817
http://speechlab.coms.uconn.edu/
Program Offerings: **i, iii, iv, v, vi, vii**

## DISTRICT OF COLUMBIA

GALLAUDET UNIVERSITY
Department of Audiology & Speech-Language
   Pathology
(202) 651-5329
http://www.gallaudet.edu/~aslpweb
Program Offerings: **i, v, vi**

GEORGE WASHINGTON UNIVERSITY
Department of Speech & Hearing Science
(202) 994-7362
http://www.gwu.edu/~sphr/
Program Offerings: **i, iii, v**

HOWARD UNIVERSITY
Department of Communication Sciences
   & Disorders
(202) 806-6990
http://www.howard.edu/
   schoolcommunications/
Program Offerings: **i, iii, iv, v, vii, x, xi**

UNIVERSITY OF THE DISTRICT OF COLUMBIA
Department of Languages & Communication
   Disorders
(202) 274-5557
http://www.udc.edu
Program Offerings: **i, iii, v, x, xi**

## FLORIDA

FLORIDA ATLANTIC UNIVERSITY
Communication Sciences & Disorders
   Program
(561) 297-2258
http://www.fau.edu
Program Offerings: **i, iv**

FLORIDA INTERNATIONAL UNIVERSITY
Communication Sciences and
   Disorders
(305) 348-2710
http://csd.fiu.edu
Program Offerings: **i, iv**

FLORIDA STATE UNIVERSITY
Department of Communication
   Disorders
(850) 644-2238
http://www.comm.fsu.edu
Program Offerings: **i, iii, iv, vii**

NOVA SOUTHEASTERN UNIVERSITY
   (SPEECH-LANGUAGE PATHOLOGY)
Speech-Language and Communication
   Disorders
(954) 262-7717
http://www.fgse.nova.edu
Program Offerings: **i, iii, iv, ix**

NOVA SOUTHEASTERN UNIVERSITY
   (AUDIOLOGY)
Audiology Department
(954) 262-7717
http://www.nova.edu
Program Offerings: **i, vi**

UNIVERSITY OF CENTRAL FLORIDA
Department of Communicative
   Disorders
(407) 823-4798
http://www.graduate.ucf.edu
Program Offerings: **i, iii, v**

UNIVERSITY OF FLORIDA
Department of Communication Sciences
   & Disorders
(352) 392-2113
http://web.csd.ufl.edu
Program Offerings: **i, iii, v, vi, vii**

UNIVERSITY OF SOUTH FLORIDA
Department of Communication Sciences &
  Disorders
(813) 974-2006
http://www.cas.usf.edu/csd/index.htm
Program Offerings: **i, iii, iv, v, vi, vii**

## GEORGIA

ARMSTRONG ATLANTIC STATE UNIVERSITY
Special Education/Speech-Language
  Pathology Program
(912) 921-7319
http://www.education.armstrong.edu/sped/
  speechlangpath.htm
Program Offerings: **i, iii, v**

GEORGIA STATE UNIVERSITY
Communication Disorders Program
(404) 651-2310
http://communication.gsu.edu
Program Offerings: **i, iii, v**

UNIVERSITY OF GEORGIA
Department of Communication Sciences
  & Disorders
(706) 542-4561
http://www.uga.edu
Program Offerings: **i, iii, iv, v**

VALDOSTA STATE UNIVERSITY
Department of Special Education
(229) 333-5932
http://coefaculty.valdosta.edu/comd/
Program Offerings: **i, iii, v**

## HAWAII

UNIVERSITY OF HAWAII AT MANOA
Department of Speech Pathology & Audiology
(808) 956-8279
http://www.hawaii.edu/spauh/
Program Offerings: **i, iii, iv, v**

## IDAHO

IDAHO STATE UNIVERSITY
Communication Sciences & Disorders, and
  Education of the Deaf
(208) 236-2196
http://www.isu.edu/departments/spchpath/
Program Offerings: **i, iii, iv, v**

## ILLINOIS

AUGUSTANA COLLEGE
Communication Sciences and Disorders
(309) 794-7350
http://www.augustana.edu
Program Offerings: **ii, iii**

EASTERN ILLINOIS UNIVERSITY
Communication Disorders & Sciences
(217) 581-2712
http://www.eiu.edu
Program Offerings: **i, iii, v**

ELMHURST COLLEGE
Communication Arts and Sciences
(630) 617-3500
http://elmhurst.edu/academics/
  academics2/?keyword=speech
Program Offerings: **ii, iii**

GOVERNORS STATE UNIVERSITY
Program in Communication Disorders
(708) 534-4590
http://www.govst.edu/cdis/
Program Offerings: **i, iii, v**

ILLINOIS STATE UNIVERSITY
Department of Speech Pathology & Audiology
(309) 438-8643
http://www.speechpathaud.ilstu.edu/
Program Offerings: **i, iii, iv, v**

NORTHERN ILLINOIS UNIVERSITY
Department of Communicative Disorders
(815) 753-1484
http://www.chhs.niu.edu/comd/
Program Offerings: **i, iii, v, vi**

NORTHWESTERN UNIVERSITY
Communication Sciences & Disorders
(847) 491-3066
http://www.northwestern.edu/csd
Program Offerings: **i, iii, iv, v, vi**

RUSH UNIVERSITY
Rush-Presbyterian-St. Luke's Medical
  Center/College of Health Sciences
Department of Communication Disorders
  & Sciences
(312) 942-6864
http://www.rushu.rush.edu/cds/
  communications.html
Program Offerings: **i, iv, v, vi**

SAINT XAVIER UNIVERSITY
Communicative Science & Disorders
(773) 298-3561
http://www.sxu.edu/comm_sci/grad/
index.html
Program Offerings: **i, iii, v**

SOUTHERN ILLINOIS UNIVERSITY
AT CARBONDALE
Communication Sciences & Disorders
(618) 453-8262
http://www.coe.siu.edu/cds/
Program Offerings: **i, iii, v**

SOUTHERN ILLINOIS UNIVERSITY AT
EDWARDSVILLE
Department of Special Education and
Communication Disorders
(618) 650-5423
http://www.siue.edu/EDUCATION/
special_ed/speech.html
Program Offerings: **i, iii, v**

UNIVERSITY OF ILLINOIS AT
URBANA-CHAMPAIGN
Department of Speech & Hearing Science
(217) 333-2230
http://www.shs.uiuc.edu/
Program Offerings: **i, iii, iv, v, vi, vii, x**

WESTERN ILLINOIS UNIVERSITY
Program in Communication Sciences and
Disorders
(309) 298-1955 ext: 241
http://www.wiu.edu/comm/
Program Offerings: **i, iii, v**

## INDIANA

BALL STATE UNIVERSITY
Department of Speech Pathology & Audiology
(765) 285-8160
http://www.bsu.edu/spaa/
Program Offerings: **i, v, vi**

BUTLER UNIVERSITY
Communication Disorders
(317) 940-9359
http://www.butler.edu/comstudies/area/
slp.html
Program Offerings: **ii, iii**

INDIANA STATE UNIVERSITY
Department of Communication Disorders and
Special Education
(812) 237-2800
http://www.indstate.edu
Program Offerings: **i, iii, v**

INDIANA UNIVERSITY
Department of Speech & Hearing Sciences
(812) 855-4156
http://www.indiana.edu/~sphsDepartment
Program Offerings: **i, iv, v, vi, vii**

PURDUE UNIVERSITY
Department of Audiology & Speech Sciences
(765) 494-3789
http://www.sla.purdue.edu/academic/aus
Program Offerings: **i, iv, v, vi, vii**

INDIANA UNIVERSITY – PURDUE
UNIVERSITY AT FORT WAYNE
Speech and Hearing Therapy
(260) 481-6410
http://www.ipfw.edu/academics/programs/s/
speech/
Program Offerings: **ii, iii**

## IOWA

UNIVERSITY OF IOWA
Department of Speech Pathology & Audiology
(319) 335-8718
http://www.shc.uiowa.edu/
Program Offerings: **i, iii, iv, v, vi, vii**

UNIVERSITY OF NORTHERN IOWA
Department of Communicative Disorders
(319) 273-2577
http://www.uni.edu/comdis/
Program Offerings: **i, iii, v**

## KANSAS

FORT HAYS STATE UNIVERSITY
Department of Communication Disorders
(785) 628-5366
http://www.fhsu.edu/commdis/
Program Offerings: **i, iii, v**

KANSAS STATE UNIVERSITY
Department of Communication Science
& Disorders
(785) 532-6879
http://courses.k-state.edu/catalog/
undergraduate/as/spch.html
Program Offerings: **i, v**

UNIVERSITY OF KANSAS
Intercampus Program in Communicative
Disorders
Department Speech, Language, Hearing
Sciences & Disorders
(913) 588-5937
http://www.lsi.ukans.edu/ipcd
Program Offerings: **i, iii, iv, v, vi, vii, x**

WICHITA STATE UNIVERSITY
Department of Communicative Disorders
& Sciences
(316) 978-3240
http://www.wichita.edu
Program Offerings: **ii, iii, iv, v, vi, vii**

# KENTUCKY

BRESCIA UNIVERSITY
Preprofessional Program in Communication
Sciences and Disorders
(270) 685-3131
http://www.brescia.edu/academics/
preprof.htm
Progam Offerings: **ii, iii**

EASTERN KENTUCKY UNIVERSITY
Department of Special Education
(859) 622-4442
http://www.education.eku.edu/Sed/CD/
Program Offerings: **i, iii, v**

MURRAY STATE UNIVERSITY
Division of Communication Disorders
(270) 762-2446
http://www.mursuky.edu
Program Offerings: **i, iii, v**

UNIVERSITY OF KENTUCKY
Division of Communication Disorders
(859) 323-1100
http://www.uky.edu
Program Offerings: **i, iii, v, vii**

UNIVERSITY OF LOUISVILLE
Division of Communicative Disorders
(502) 852-5274
http://www.louisville.edu/medschool/
surgery/com_disorders
Program Offerings: **i, v, vi**

WESTERN KENTUCKY UNIVERSITY
Communication Disorders Program
(270) 745-4302
http://www.wku.edu/Department/Academic/
chhs/commdis/
Program Offerings: **i, iii, v**

# LOUISIANA

GRAMBLING STATE UNIVERSITY
Speech and Hearing Clinic
(318) 274-2344
http://www.gram.edu/Colleges_Schools/
Liberal%20Arts/Speech%20&%20Theatre
/index.htm
Program Offerings: **ii, iii, xi**

LOUISIANA STATE UNIVERSITY AND A&M
COLLEGE
Division of Communication Sciences
& Disorders
(225) 578-2545
http://www.lsu.edu
Program Offerings: **i, iii, iv, v**

LOUISIANA STATE UNIVERSITY HEALTH
SCIENCES CENTER IN NEW ORLEANS
Department of Communication Disorders
(504) 568-4348
http://www.lsuhsc.edu/
Program Offerings: **i, iv, v, vi, vii**

LOUISIANA STATE UNIVERSITY HEALTH
SCIENCES CENTER IN SHREVEPORT
Department of Rehabilitation Sciences
(318) 632-2015
http://www.sh.lsuhsc.edu/ah/
Program Offerings: **i, v**

LOUISIANA TECH UNIVERSITY
Department of Speech
(318) 257-4764
http://www.latech.edu/tech/liberal-arts/
speech/Degrees/MASLPA.html
Program Offerings: **i, iii, iv, v, vi**

NICHOLLS STATE UNIVERSITY
Department of Allied Health Sciences
(985) 448-4585
http://www.nicholls.edu/acad/
    bulletin01-02/bltnalhe.html#comm
Program Offerings: **ii, iii**

SOUTHEASTERN LOUISIANA UNIVERSITY
Department of Communication Sciences
    & Disorders
(985) 549-2214
http://www.selu.edu/Academics/Nursing/
    csd/
Program Offerings: **i, iii, v**

SOUTHERN UNIVERSITY AND A&M COLLEGE
Communication Disorders Program
(225) 771-3950
http://www.subr.edu
Program Offerings: **i, iii, v**

UNIVERSITY OF LOUISIANA AT LAFAYETTE
Department of Communicative Disorders
(337) 482-6721
http://www.louisiana.edu/Academic/
    LiberalArts/CODI/
Program Offerings: **i, iii, v**

UNIVERSITY OF LOUISIANA AT MONROE
Department of Communicative Disorders
(318) 342-3192
http://www.ulm.edu/codi/
Program Offerings: **i, iii, v**

XAVIAR UNIVERSITY OF LOUISIANA
Department of Education
(504) 520-7536
http://www.xula.edu/education/
Program Offerings: **ii, iii, xi**

## MAINE

UNIVERSITY OF MAINE AT ORONO
Department of Communication Sciences
    & Disorders
(207) 581-2006
http://www.umaine.edu/comscidis/
Program Offerings: **i, iii, v**

## MARYLAND

LOYOLA COLLEGE IN MARYLAND
Department of Speech-Language Pathology
(410) 617-7623
http://www.loyola.edu
Program Offerings: **i, iii, v**

TOWSON UNIVERSITY
Department of Communication Sciences
    & Disorders
(410) 704-4153
http://www.towson.edu/~wgabbay/
    csd_hpg.html
Program Offerings: **i, iii, iv, v, vi**

UNIVERSITY OF MARYLAND, COLLEGE PARK
Department of Hearing & Speech Sciences
(301) 405-4214
http://www.bsos.umd.edu/hesp/
Program Offerings: **i, iii, iv, v, vi, vii**

## MASSACHUSETTS

BOSTON UNIVERSITY
Programs in Communication Disorders
Department of Health Sciences
(617) 353-3188
http://www.bu.edu/sargent/cd
Program Offerings: **i, iii, v, viii**

BRIDGEWATER STATE COLLEGE
Department of Special Education
(508) 531-1000
http://www.bridgew.edu/Programs.cfm
Program Offerings: **ii, iii**

ELMS COLLEGE
Division of Health Sciences
(413) 594-2761 ext. 237
http://www.elms.edu/academics/
    undergraduate/health.htm
Program Offerings: **ii, iii**

EMERSON COLLEGE
Department of Communication Sciences
    & Disorders
(617) 824-8730
http://www.emerson.edu/communication_
    disorders/
Program Offerings: **i, iii, v, vii**

MGH INSTITUTE OF HEALTH PROFESSIONS
Graduate Program in Communication
    Sciences & Disorders
(617) 726-8019
http://www.mghihp.edu/Academics/
    Comm.html
Program Offerings: **i, v**

NORTHEASTERN UNIVERSITY
Department of Speech-Language Pathology
    & Audiology
(617) 373-3698
http://www.bouve.neu.edu/Graduate/Health/
    communication_slp.html
Program Offerings: **i, iii, iv, v**

SALEM STATE COLLEGE
Theater and Speech Communications
(978) 542-6000
http://www.salemstate.edu/theatre_speech/
    TSC-speech_communication.php
Program Offerings: **ii, iii**

UNIVERSITY OF MASSACHUSETTS AT
    AMHERST
Department of Communication Disorders
(413) 545-0131
http://www.umass.edu/sphhs/comdis/
    graduate.html
Program Offerings: **i, iii, iv, v, vii**

WORCESTER STATE COLLEGE
Communication Sciences and Disorders
(508) 929-8055
http://www.worcester.edu/academics/comm
    _disorders/master_comm_disorders.htm
Program Offerings: **i, iii, v**

# MICHIGAN

ANDREWS UNIVERSITY
Speech-Language Pathology And Audiology
(269) 471-3468
http://www.andrews.edu/academic/cas/
    speech_path.php3
Program Offerings: **ii, iii**

CALVIN COLLEGE
Communication Arts and Sciences
(616) 526-6283
http://www.calvin.edu/academic/cas/
    programs/speech/index.htm
Program Offerings: **ii, iii**

CENTRAL MICHIGAN UNIVERSITY
Department of Communication Disorders
(989) 774-3803
http://www.chp.cmich.edu/cdo.
Program Offerings: **i, iii, vi**

EASTERN MICHIGAN UNIVERSITY
Speech Language Impaired Program
(734) 487-3300
http://www.emich.edu/coe/speced/
Program Offerings: **i, iii, v**

MICHIGAN STATE UNIVERSITY
Department of Audiology & Speech Sciences
(517) 353-8780
http://asc.msu.edu/
Program Offerings: **i, iii, iv, v, vii**

NORTHERN MICHIGAN UNIVERSITY
Department of Communication Disorders
(906) 227-2125
http://www.nmu.edu/departments/
    commdisorders.htm
Program Offerings: **i, iii, v**

WAYNE STATE UNIVERSITY
Audiology & Speech-Language Pathology
(313) 577-3339
http://www.science.wayne.edu/~aslp
Program Offerings: **i, iii, v, vi, vii**

WESTERN MICHIGAN UNIVERSITY
Department of Speech Pathology & Audiology
(616) 387-8045
http://www.wmich.edu/hhs/sppa/
Program Offerings: **i, iii, iv, v, vi**

# MINNESOTA

MINNESOTA STATE UNIVERSITY – MANKATO
Communication Disorders Program
(507) 389-1414
http://www.mnsu.edu/comdis/Departmenthp/
    comdis.html
Program Offerings: **i, iii, v**

MINNESOTA STATE UNIVERSITY –
    MOORHEAD
Department of Speech/Language/ Hearing
    Sciences
(218) 236-2286
http://www.mnstate.edu/slhs/
Program Offerings: **i, iii, v**

SAINT CLOUD STATE UNIVERSITY
Department of Communication Disorders
(320) 308-2092
http://www.stcloudstate.edu/commdisorders
Program Offerings: **i, iii, v**

UNIVERSITY OF MINNESOTA
Department of Communication Disorders
(612) 624-3322
http://www.cdis.umn.edu/
Program Offerings: **i, iii, iv, v, vi, vii, x**

UNIVERSITY OF MINNESOTA – DULUTH
Communication Disorders Program
(218) 726-7974
http://www.d.umn.edu/csd/
Program Offerings: **i, iii, v**

# MISSISSIPPI

DELTA STATE UNIVERSITY
Department of Audiology-Speech Pathology
(662) 846-4110
http://www.deltastate.edu/academics/artsci/
    audsp/index.html
Program Offerings: **ii, iii**

JACKSON STATE UNIVERSITY
Department of Communicative Disorders
(601) 432-6713
http://www.jsums.edu/liberalarts/sda/
    commdisorders.htm
Program Offerings: **i, iii, v**

MISSISSIPPI UNIVERSITY FOR WOMEN
Speech-Language Pathology/Audiology
(662) 329-7270
http://www.muw.edu/speech_hear/slp.htm
Program Offerings: **i, iii, v**

UNIVERSITY OF MISSISSIPPI
Department of Communicative Disorders
(662) 915-7652
http://www.olemiss.edu/Departments/
    comm_disorders/
Program Offerings: **i, iii, v**

UNIVERSITY OF SOUTHERN MISSISSIPPI
Department of Speech & Hearing Sciences
(601) 266-5216
http://www.usm.edu/shs/
Program Offerings: **i, iii, iv, v, vi**

# MISSOURI

CENTRAL MISSOURI STATE UNIVERSITY
Department of Communication Disorders
(660) 543-4993
http://comdisorders.cmsu.edu/
Program Offerings: **i, iii, iv, v**

FONTBONNE UNIVERSITY
Department of Communication Disorders and
    Deaf Education
(314) 889-1407
http://www.fontbonne.edu
Program Offerings: **i, iii, v**

ROCKHURST UNIVERSITY
Communication Sciences & Disorders
(816) 501-4255
http://www.rockhurst.edu/admission/grad/
    csd/index.asp
Program Offerings: **i, iii, v**

SAINT LOUIS UNIVERSITY
Communication Sciences & Disorders
(314) 977-2940
http://www.slu.edu/colleges/cops/cd/
Program Offerings: **i, iii, v, x**

SOUTHEAST MISSOURI STATE UNIVERSITY
Department of Communication Disorders
(573) 651-2155
http://www.semo.edu/study/commdisorders/
    index.htm
Program Offerings: **i, iii, v**

SOUTHWEST MISSOURI STATE UNIVERSITY
Department of Communication Sciences
    and Disorders
(417) 836-5368
http://www.smsu.edu/CSD/
Program Offerings: **i, iii, iv, v, vi**

TRUMAN STATE UNIVERSITY
Department of Communication Disorders
(660) 785-4675
http://www2.truman.edu/comdis/
Program Offerings: **i, iii, v**

UNIVERSITY OF MISSOURI, COLUMBIA
Department of Communication Science
    & Disorders
(573) 882-3873
http://www.umshp.org/csd/
Program Offerings: **ii, iii, v, vii**

WASHINGTON UNIVERSITY
Program in Audiology and Communication
    Sciences
(314) 977-0240
http://www.cid.wustl.edu/
Program Offerings: **i, v, vi, vii**

## NEBRASKA

UNIVERSITY OF NEBRASKA, KEARNEY
Communication Disorders Program
(308) 865-8300
http://www.unk.edu/acad/cdis/home.html
Program Offerings: **i, iii, v**

UNIVERSITY OF NEBRASKA, LINCOLN
Department of Special Education &
    Communication Disorders
(402) 472-5496
http://www.unl.edu/barkley/comdis/
    index.html
Program Offerings: **i, iii, iv, v, vii**

UNIVERSITY OF NEBRASKA, OMAHA
Special Education & Communication
    Disorders
(402) 554-2201
http://www.unocoe.unomaha.edu/sped.htm
Program Offerings: **i, iii, v**

## NEVADA

UNIVERSITY OF NEVADA, RENO
Department of Speech Pathology & Audiology
(775) 784-4887
http://www.unr.edu/spa/
Program Offerings: **i, iii, v, vii**

## NEW HAMPSHIRE

UNIVERSITY OF NEW HAMPSHIRE
Department of Communication Sciences and
    Disorders
(603) 862-2125
http://www.shhs.unh.edu/csd/
Program Offerings: **i, iii, v**

## NEW JERSEY

KEAN UNIVERSITY
Department of Communication Disorders and
    Deafness

(908) 527-2218
http://www.kean.edu/~keangrad/
    grad_CE_slp.htm
Program Offerings: **i, iii, v**

MONTCLAIR STATE UNIVERSITY
Department of Communication Sciences
    & Disorders
(973) 655-4232
http://www.chss.montclair.edu/csd/csd.htm
Program Offerings: **i, v**

RICHARD STOCKTON COLLEGE OF
    NEW JERSEY
Speech Pathology and Audiology
(609) 652-4501
http://www2.Stockton.edu
Program Offerings: **ii, iii**

SETON HALL UNIVERSITY
School of Graduate Medical Education
Department of Speech-Language Pathology
    and Audiology
(973) 275-2825
http://gradmeded.shu.edu
Program Offerings: **i, v, vii, ix**

THE COLLEGE OF NEW JERSEY
Language & Communication Sciences
(609) 771-2399
http://www.tcnj.edu
Program Offerings: **i, iii, v**

WILLIAM PATERSON UNIVERSITY
Department of Communication Disorders
(973) 720-2208
http://www.wpunj.edu/cos/comm-disorders/
Program Offerings: **i, iii, v**

## NEW MEXICO

EASTERN NEW MEXICO UNIVERSITY
Department of Communicative Disorders
(505) 562-2156
http://www.enmu.edu
Program Offerings: **i, iii, v**

NEW MEXICO STATE UNIVERSITY
Department of Special Education/
    Communication Disorders
(505) 646-2402
http://education.nmsu.edu/sped/
Program Offerings: **i, iii, v, x**

UNIVERSITY OF NEW MEXICO
Department of Speech & Hearing Sciences
(505) 277-4453
http://www.unm.edu/~sphrsci/
Program Offerings: **i, iii, v**

# NEW YORK

ADELPHI UNIVERSITY
Communication Sciences & Disorders
(516) 877-4770
http://www.academics.adelphi.edu/edu/csd/
Program Offerings: **i, iii, iv, v, ix**

BROOKLYN COLLEGE OF CUNY
Speech-Language Pathology & Audiology
(718) 951-5186
http://www.brooklyn.cuny.edu/apiindex.htm
Program Offerings: **i, iii, iv, v**

BUFFALO STATE COLLEGE
Department of Speech-Language Pathology
(716) 878-5719
http://www.buffalostate.edu/depts/speech
Program Offerings: **i, iii, v**

COLLEGE OF SAINT ROSE
Communication Disorders Department
(518) 454-5236
http://www.strose.edu
Program Offerings: **i, iii, v**

ELMIRA COLLEGE
Speech and Hearing
(607) 735-1800
http://www.elmira.edu
Program Offerings: **ii, iii**

HOFSTRA UNIVERSITY
Department of Speech-Language-Hearing
  Sciences
(516) 463-5508
http://www.hofstra.edu
Program Offerings: **i, iii, iv, v**

HUNTER COLLEGE OF CUNY
Communication Sciences Program
(212) 481-4467
http://www.hunter.cuny.edu/schoolhp/
  comsc/index.htm
Program Offerings: **i, iv, v, vi**

IONA COLLEGE
Speech Communication Studies
(914) 633-2168
http://www.iona.edu
Program Offerings: **ii, iii**

ITHACA COLLEGE
Speech-Language Pathology & Audiology
(607) 274-3248
http://www.ithaca.edu/hshp/slpa/
  DEPARTMENTHOMEPAGE/
Program Offerings: **i, iii, v**

LEHMAN COLLEGE OF CUNY
Speech-Language-Hearing Sciences
(718) 960-8138
http://www.lehman.cuny.edu/
Program Offerings: **i, iii, v**

LONG ISLAND UNIVERSITY, BROOKLYN
  CAMPUS
Communication Sciences and Disorders
(718) 488-4007
http://www.brooklyn.liu.edu/
Program Offerings: **i, iii, v, x**

LONG ISLAND UNIVERSITY, C.W.
  POST CAMPUS
Communication Sciences and Disorders
(516) 299-2436
http://www.cwpost.liu.edu/cwis/cwp/edu/
  speehear/speehear.html
Program Offerings: **i, iii, v**

MARYMOUNT MANHATTAN COLLEGE
Division of Sciences
(212) 774-0720
http://marymount.mmm.edu
Program Offerings: **ii, iii**

MERCY COLLEGE
Communication Disorders Department
(914) 674-7421
http://grad.mercy.edu/commdisorder/
  index.htm
Program Offerings: **i, iii, v**

NAZARETH COLLEGE OF ROCHESTER
Department of Communication Sciences
  and Disorders
(585) 389-2773
http://www.naz.edu/dept/speech/
Program Offerings: **i, iii, v, x**

NEW YORK MEDICAL COLLEGE
Speech-Language Pathology
(914) 594-4239
http://www.nymc.edu/sph/programs/SLP/
Program Offerings: **i, v**

NEW YORK UNIVERSITY
Speech-Language Pathology & Audiology
(212) 998-5230
http://www.nyu.edu/education/speech/
Program Offerings: **i, iii, v, vii**

PLATTSBURGH STATE UNIVERSITY OF
NEW YORK
Communication Disorders and Sciences
(518) 564-2170
http://spectra.plattsburgh.edu/cds/
Program Offerings: **i, iii, v**

QUEENS COLLEGE OF CUNY
Department of Linguistics & Communication
Disorders
(718) 997-2930
http://qcpages.qc.edu/LCD/
Program Offerings: **i, iii, v, vii**

SAINT JOHN'S UNIVERSITY
Grad. Program in Speech-Language Pathology
& Audiology
(718) 990-6480
http://new.stjohns.edu/
Program Offerings: **i, iv, v, x**

STATE UNIVERSITY OF NEW YORK
AT BUFFALO
Communicative Disorders & Sciences
(716) 829-2797
http://wings.buffalo.edu/cds/
Program Offerings: **i, iii, v, vi, vii**

STATE UNIVERSITY OF NEW YORK
AT CORTLAND
Speech Pathology and Audiology Department
(607) 756-5423
http://www.cortland.edu/spchpath/
Program Offerings: **ii, iii**

STATE UNIVERSITY OF NEW YORK
AT NEW PALTZ
Department of Communication Disorders
(845) 257-3620
http://www.newpaltz.edu/commdis
Program Offerings: **i, iii, iv, v**

STATE UNIVERSITY OF NEW YORK, COLLEGE
AT FREDONIA
Department of Speech Pathology & Audiology
(716) 673-3202
http://www.fredonia.edu/gradstudies/
msspeechpath.htm
Program Offerings: **i, iii, v**

STATE UNIVERSITY OF NEW YORK, COLLEGE
AT GENESEO
Department of Communicative Disorders &
Sciences
(585) 245-5328
http://www.geneseo.edu
Program Offerings: **i, iii, v**

STERN COLLEGE FOR WOMEN-YESHIVA
UNIVERSITY
Speech Pathology & Audiology
(212) 340-7701
http://www.yu.edu/stern/speechpathology/
Program Offerings: **ii, iii**

SYRACUSE UNIVERSITY
Department of Communication Sciences
& Disorders
(315) 443-9637
http://thecollege.syr.edu/Departments/csd/
Program Offerings: **i, iii, iv, v, vi, vii**

TEACHERS COLLEGE, COLUMBIA UNIVERSITY
Speech and Language Pathology and
Audiology
(212) 678-3895
http://www.tc.edu/academic/bbs/
speech-language/
Program Offerings: **i, iii, v, x**

TOURO COLLEGE
Department of Speech
(718) 252-7800
http://www.touro.edu/gsp/
Program Offerings: **i, iii, v**

## NORTH CAROLINA

APPALACHIAN STATE UNIVERSITY
Department of Language, Reading &
Exceptionalities
(828) 262-2182
http://www.lre.appstate.edu/
Program Offerings: **i, iii, v**

EAST CAROLINA UNIVERSITY
Department of Communication Sciences &
 Disorders
(252) 328-4404
http://www.ecu.edu/csd/
Program Offerings: **i, iii, iv, v, vi, vii**

ELIZABETH CITY STATE UNIVERSITY
Language, Literature and Communication
 Department
(252) 335-3349
http://www.ecsu.edu/curriculum/speech-
 path.cfm
Program Offerings: **ii, iii, xi**

NORTH CAROLINA A & T STATE UNIVERSITY
Speech Pathology & Audiology
(336) 334-7806
http://www.ncat.edu
Program Offerings: **iii, xi**

NORTH CAROLINA CENTRAL UNIVERSITY
Department of Communication Disorders
(919) 530-7473
http://www.nccu.edu
Program Offerings: **i, v**

NORTH CAROLINA STATE UNIVERSITY
Communication Department
(919) 515-2011
http://www.ncsu.edu
Program Offerings: **ii, iii**

SHAW UNIVERSITY
Department of Allied Health Professions,
 Speech Pathology and Audiology
(919) 546-8373
http://www.shawu.edu
Program Offerings: **ii, iii, xi**

UNIVERSITY OF NORTH CAROLINA AT
 CHAPEL HILL
Division of Speech & Hearing Sciences
(919) 966-1006
http://www.med.unc.edu/ahs/sphs
Program Offerings: **i, v, vi, vii**

UNIVERSITY OF NORTH CAROLINA AT
 GREENSBORO
Communication Sciences & Disorders
(336) 334-5184
http://www.uncg.edu/csd/
Program Offerings: **i, iii, iv, v**

WESTERN CAROLINA UNIVERSITY
Human Services
(828) 227-7310
http://www.wcu.edu/graduate/
 communicationdisorders.html
Program Offerings: **i, iii, v**

## NORTH DAKOTA

MINOT STATE UNIVERSITY
Department of Communication Disorders and
 Special Education
(701) 858-3031
http://www.minotstateu.edu/cdse/
Program Offerings: **i, iii, iv, v**

UNIVERSITY OF NORTH DAKOTA
Communication Sciences & Disorders
(701) 777-3232
http://www.und.edu/Department/cdis/
 index.html
Program Offerings: **i, iii, v**

## OHIO

BALDWIN-WALLACE COLLEGE
Communication Disorders
(440) 826-2900
http://www.bw.edu/academics/comdis/
Program Offerings: **ii, iii**

BOWLING GREEN STATE UNIVERSITY
Department of Communication Disorders
(419) 372-2515
http://www.bgsu.edu/departments/cdis/
Program Offerings: **i, iii, v, vii**

CASE WESTERN RESERVE UNIVERSITY
Department of Communication Sciences
(216) 368-2556
http://www.cwru.edu/artsci/cosi/
Program Offerings: **i, iii, v, vii**

CLEVELAND STATE UNIVERSITY
Department of Speech & Hearing
(216) 687-6986
http://www.csuohio.edu
Program Offerings: **i, iii, v**

COLLEGE OF WOOSTER
Department of Communication
(330) 263-6000
http://www.wooster.edu
Program Offerings: **ii, iii**

KENT STATE UNIVERSITY
School of Speech Pathology & Audiology
(330) 672-2672
http://dept.kent.edu/spa/
Program Offerings: **i, iii, v, vi, vii**

MIAMI UNIVERSITY
Department of Speech Pathology and
   Audiology
(513) 529-2500
http://www.miami.muohio.edu
Program Offerings: **i, iii, iv, v**

OHIO STATE UNIVERSITY
Department of Speech & Hearing Science
(614) 292-8207
http://www.acs.ohio-state.edu/sphs/
Program Offerings: **i, iii, iv, v, vii**

OHIO UNIVERSITY
School of Hearing, Speech and Language
   Sciences
(740) 593-1407
http://www.ohiou.edu/hearingspeech/
   index.htm
Program Offerings: **i, iii, v, vi, vii**

UNIVERSITY OF AKRON - NORTHEAST OHIO
   AUDIOLOGY CONSORTIUM
   (U. Akron/Kent State U.)
School of Speech Pathology and Audiology
(330) 972-6119
http://www.uakron.edu/index.php
Program Offerings: **i, vi**

UNIVERSITY OF AKRON
School of Speech-Language & Audiology
(330) 972-6803
http://www.uakron.edu/colleges/faa/depts/
   sslpa/
Program Offerings: **i, iii, v, vi**

UNIVERSITY OF CINCINNATI
Communication Sciences & Disorders
(513) 558-8501
http://www.uc.edu/csd
Program Offerings: **i, iii, iv, v, vi, vii**

UNIVERSITY OF TOLEDO
Public Health and Rehabilitative Services
(419) 530-8473
http://www.hhs.utoledo.edu/speech/
   graduateprogram.html
Program Offerings: **i, iii, v**

## OKLAHOMA

NORTHEASTERN STATE UNIVERSITY
Speech-Language Pathology Program
(918) 456-5511
http://arapaho.nsuok.edu/%7Ecollegeofed/
   speech_path/index.htm
Program Offerings: **i, iii, v**

OKLAHOMA STATE UNIVERSITY
Department of Communication Sciences
   & Disorders
(405) 744-6021
http://www.cas.okstate.edu/cdis/
Program Offerings: **i, iii, v**

UNIVERSITY OF CENTRAL OKLAHOMA
Department of Curriculum & Instruction
(405) 974-5297
http://www.ucok.edu
Program Offerings: **i, v**

UNIVERSITY OF OKLAHOMA HEALTH
   SCIENCES CENTER
Department of Communication Sciences
   & Disorders
(405) 271-4214
http://www.ouhsc.edu/ahealth/faccsd.htm
Program Offerings: **i, iii, v, vi, vii, xii**

UNIVERSITY OF SCIENCES & ARTS
   OF OKLAHOMA
Division of Education and Speech-Language
   Pathology
(405) 224-3140
http://www.usao.edu
Program Offerings: **ii, iii**

UNIVERSITY OF TULSA
Department of Communication Disorders
(918) 631-2504
http://www.cas.utulsa.edu/commdis/
Program Offerings: **i, iii, v**

## OREGON

PORTLAND STATE UNIVERSITY
Speech & Hearing Sciences Program
(503) 725-3533
http://www.sphr.pdx.edu
Program Offerings: **i, iii, iv, v**

UNIVERSITY OF OREGON
Communication Disorders & Sciences
Program
(541) 346-2480
http://education.uoregon.edu
Program Offerings: **i, iii, v, vii**

## PENNSYLVANIA

BLOOMSBURG UNIVERSITY
Department of Audiology & Speech Pathology
(570) 389-4436
http://www.bloomu.edu/academic/aud/
Program Offerings: **i, iii, iv, v, vi**

CALIFORNIA UNIVERSITY OF PENNSYLVANIA
Department of Communication Disorders
(724) 938-4175
http://www.cup.edu/ugcatalog/Programs/
CommDisorders.htm
Program Offerings: **i, iii, v**

CLARION UNIVERSITY OF PENNSYLVANIA
Department of Communication Sciences
& Disorders
(814) 393-2581
http://www.clarion.edu/departments/csd/
Program Offerings: **i, iii, v**

COLLEGE MISERICORDIA
Department of Speech-Language Pathology
(570) 674-6471
http://www.miseri.edu/academics/
healthweb/SpeechLanguage/index.htm
Program Offerings: **i, iii, v**

DUQUESNE UNIVERSITY
Department of Speech-Language Pathology
(412) 396-4225
http://www.slp.duq.edu/
Program Offerings: **i, v**

EAST STROUDSBURG UNIVERSITY OF PENN-
SYLVANIA
Department of Speech Pathology & Audiology
(570) 422-3247
http://www3.esu.edu/academics/hshp/sppa/
home.asp
Program Offerings: **i, iii, v**

EDINBORO UNIVERSITY OF PENNSYLVANIA
Speech & Communication Studies/Speech-
Language Pathology
(814) 732-2432

http://www.edinboro.edu
Program Offerings: **i, iii, v**

GENEVA COLLEGE
Communication Disorders
(724) 846-5100
http://www.geneva.edu
Program Offerings: **ii, iii**

INDIANA UNIVERSITY OF PENNSYLVANIA
Special Education & Clinical Svcs-Speech-
Language Pathology Program
(724) 357-2450
http://www.iup.edu/special-ed/
Program Offerings: **i, iii, v**

KUTZTOWN UNIVERSITY
Special Education Department
(610) 683-4290
http://www.kutztown.edu
Program Offerings: **ii, iii**

LA SALLE UNIVERSITY
Speech-Language-Hearing Sciences Program
(215) 951-1986
http://www.lasalle.edu/academ/grad/slhs/
slhs.htm
Program Offerings: **i, iii, v**

MARYWOOD UNIVERSITY
Communication Sciences & Disorders
(570) 348-6299
http://www.marywood.edu/departments/
commsci/csdpage.stm
Program Offerings: **i, iii, v**

PENNSYLVANIA COLLEGE OF OPTOMETRY
Audiology Department
(215) 780-1238
http://www.AuDonline.org
Program Offerings: **i, vi**

PENNSYLVANIA STATE UNIVERSITY
Communication Sciences and Disorders
(814) 865-3177
http://www.pco.edu/acad_progs/Audiology/
aud_progrs.htm
Program Offerings: **i, iii, v, vii**

TEMPLE UNIVERSITY
Communication Sciences
(215) 204-1878
http://www.temple.edu/commsci/
Program Offerings: **i, iii, v, vii, x**

THIEL COLLEGE
Speech and Hearing Science
(724) 589-2345
http://www.thiel.edu
Program Offerings: **ii, iii**

UNIVERSITY OF PITTSBURGH
Communication Science and Disorders
(412) 383-6541
http://www.shrs.pitt.edu/csd/index.html
Program Offerings: **i, iii, iv, v, vi, vii**

WEST CHESTER UNIVERSITY
Department of Communicative Disorders
(610) 436-3401
http://www.wcupa.edu/_academics/
   sch_shs.spp/
Program Offerings: **i, iii, v**

## PUERTO RICO

UNIVERSITY OF PUERTO RICO
Speech-Language Pathology & Audiology
(787) 758-2525
http://www.upr.clu.edu/
Program Offerings: **i, iv, v**

## RHODE ISLAND

RHODE ISLAND COLLEGE
Speech & Hearing Science
(401) 456-8270
http://www.ric.edu
Program Offerings: **ii, iii**

UNIVERSITY OF RHODE ISLAND
Department of Communicative Disorders
(401) 874-5969
http://www.uri.edu/hss/cmd
Program Offerings: **i, iii, iv, v, vi**

## SOUTH CAROLINA

COLUMBIA COLLEGE
Speech-Language Pathology Program
(803) 786-3642
http://www.columbiacollegesc.edu
Program Offerings: **ii, iii**

MEDICAL UNIVERSITY OF SOUTH CAROLINA
Communication Sciences and Disorders
   Program
(843) 792-2023
http://www.musc.edu/chp/csd/
Program Offerings: **i, v**

SOUTH CAROLINA STATE UNIVERSITY
Department of Speech Pathology & Audiology
(803) 536-8074
http://www.scsu.edu/SPA/
Program Offerings: **i, iii, v**

UNIVERSITY OF SOUTH CAROLINA
Communication Sciences and Disorders
(803) 777-4813
http://www.sph.sc.edu/Comd/comdaboutus.
   asp
Program Offerings: **ii, iii, v**

WINTHROP UNIVERSITY
Department of Speech
(803) 323-2379
http://www.winthrop.edu
Program Offerings: **ii, iii**

## SOUTH DAKOTA

AUGUSTANA COLLEGE
Communication Disorders
(605) 274-0770
http://www.augie.edu
Program Offerings: **ii, iii**

UNIVERSITY OF SOUTH DAKOTA
Department of Communication Disorders
(605) 677-5474
http://www.usd.edu/dcom/
Program Offerings: **i, iii, iv, v**

## TENNESSEE

EAST TENNESSEE STATE UNIVERSITY
Department of Communicative Disorders
(423) 439-4272
http://www.etsu.edu/cpah/commdis/
   index.htm
Program Offerings: **i, iv, v, vi**

MIDDLE TENNESSEE STATE UNIVERSITY
Speech and Theatre Department
(615) 898-2640
http://www.mtsu.edu
Program Offerings: **ii, iii**

TENNESSEE STATE UNIVERSITY
Department of Speech Pathology & Audiology
(615) 963-7081
http://www.tnstate.edu/speechpath/
Program Offerings: **i, iii, v, xi**

UNIVERSITY OF MEMPHIS
School of Audiology & Speech-Language
   Pathology
(901) 678-5877
http://www.ausp.memphis.edu
Program Offerings: **i, v, vi, vii, x, xii**

UNIVERSITY OF TENNESSEE AT KNOXVILLE
Department of Audiology & Speech Pathology
(865) 974-5019
http://web.utk.edu/~aspweb/
Program Offerings: **i, iii, iv, v, vi, vii**

VANDERBILT UNIVERSITY
Division of Hearing & Speech Sciences
(615) 936-5000
http://www.vanderbilt.edu/
   BillWilkersonCenter/
Program Offerings: **i, iii, iv, v, vi, vii**

## TEXAS

ABILENE CHRISTIAN UNIVERSITY
Communication Sciences and Disorders
   Division
(915) 674-2074
http://www.acu.edu/academics/cas/comm_
   disorders.html
Program Offerings: **i, iii, v**

BAYLOR UNIVERSITY
Department of Communication Sciences
   & Disorders
(254) 710-2567
http://www.baylor.edu/communication_
   disorders/
Program Offerings: **i, iii, v**

LAMAR UNIVERSITY - BEAUMONT
Department of Communication Disorders
   & Deaf Education
(409) 880-8338
http://dept.lamar.edu/cofac/cmds/
Program Offerings: **i, iii, iv, v, vi**

OUR LADY OF THE LAKE UNIVERSITY
Program in Communication & Learning
   Disorders
(210) 434-6711
http://www.ollusa.edu/academic/secs/
   communication_disorders.html
Program Offerings: **i, iii, v**

SOUTHWEST TEXAS STATE UNIVERSITY
Department of Communication Disorders
(512) 245-2330
http://www.health.txstate.edu/CDIS/
   cdis.html
Program Offerings: **i, iii, v**

STEPHEN F. AUSTIN STATE UNIVERSITY
Speech-Language Pathology Program
(936) 468-1252
http://www.sfasu.edu/aas/comm/
Program Offerings: **i, iii, v**

TEXAS A&M UNIVERSITY, KINGSVILLE
Communication Sciences & Disorders
(361) 593-3401
http://www.tamuk.edu
Program Offerings: **i, iii, v**

TEXAS CHRISTIAN UNIVERSITY
Communication Sciences & Disorders
(817) 257-7621
http://www.csd.tcu.edu/
Program Offerings: **i, iii, v, x**

TEXAS TECH UNIVERSITY
Department of Speech, Language, and
   Hearing Sciences
(806) 743-5660
http://www.ttuhsc.edu/SAH/programs.htm
Program Offerings: **i, iii, v, vi**

TEXAS WOMAN'S UNIVERSITY
Communication Sciences & Disorders
(940) 898-2025
http://www.twu.edu/hs/comms/
Program Offerings: **i, iii, v, xii**

UNIVERSITY OF HOUSTON
Program in Communication Disorders
(713) 743-2896
http://www.class.uh.edu/comd/
Program Offerings: **i, iii, v**

UNIVERSITY OF NORTH TEXAS
Department of Speech & Hearing Sciences
(940) 565-2481
http://www.sphs.unt.edu
Program Offerings: **i, iii, iv, v, vi**

UNIVERSITY OF TEXAS AT AUSTIN
Communication Sciences & Disorders
(512) 471-4119
http://csd.utexas.edu/
Program Offerings: **i, iii, iv, v, vii, x**

UNIVERSITY OF TEXAS AT DALLAS
Program in Communication Disorders
UTD Callier Center for Communication
    Disorders
(214) 905-3060
http://www.utdallas.edu/dept/bbs/
Program Offerings: **i, iii, iv, v, vi, vii**

UNIVERSITY OF TEXAS AT EL PASO
Department of Speech-Language Pathology
(915) 747-7250
http://chs.utep.edu/slp/home.html
Program Offerings: **i, iii, v**

UNIVERSITY OF TEXAS-PAN AMERICAN
Department of Communication Sciences and
    Disorders
(956) 316-7040
http://www.panam.edu/dept/commdisorder/
Program Offerings: **i, iii, v, x**

WEST TEXAS A&M UNIVERSITY
Program in Communication Disorders
(806) 651-2799
http://www.wtamu.edu/academic/fah/art/
    comunicationdisorders.html
Program Offerings: **i, iii, v**

## UTAH

BRIGHAM YOUNG UNIVERSITY
Department of Audiology & Speech-Language
    Pathology
(801) 422-5117
http://www.byu.edu/aslp/
Program Offerings: **i, iii, iv, v**

UNIVERSITY OF UTAH
Department of Communication Sciences and
    Disorders
(801) 581-6725
http://www.health.utah.edu/cmdis/
Program Offerings: **i, iii, iv, v, vi, vii**

UTAH STATE UNIVERSITY
Department of Communicative Disorders
    & Deaf Education
(435) 797-1375
http://www.coe.usu.edu/comd/
Program Offerings: **i, iii, iv, v, vi**

## VERMONT

UNIVERSITY OF VERMONT
Communication Sciences
(802) 656-3861
http://www.uvm.edu/~cmsi/
Program Offerings: **i, iii, v**

## VIRGINIA

HAMPTON UNIVERSITY
Department of Communicative Sciences
    & Disorders
(757) 727-5435
http://www.hamptonu.edu/science/
    communicativedisorders/masters.htm
Program Offerings: **i, iv**

JAMES MADISON UNIVERSITY
Communication Sciences & Disorders
(540) 568-6440
http://www.csd.jmu.edu/
Program Offerings: **i, iii, iv, v, vi, vii**

LONGWOOD COLLEGE
Dept. of Education, Special Education, and
    Social Work – Communication Disorders
(434) 395-2771
http://www.lwc.edu
Program Offerings: **ii, iii**

NORFOLK STATE UNIVERSITY
Communication Sciences and Disorders
    Program
(757) 823-9430
http://www.nsu.edu/schools/liberalarts/enfl/
    programs.html
Program Offerings: **ii, iii, xi**

OLD DOMINION UNIVERSITY
Speech-Language Pathology
(757) 683-4117
web.odu.edu/esse
Program Offerings: **i, iii, v**

RADFORD UNIVERSITY
Department of Communication Sciences
    & Disorders
(540) 831-7666
http://www.radford.edu/~cosd-web/
Program Offerings: **i, iii, v**

UNIVERSITY OF VIRGINIA
Communication Disorders Program
(434) 924-7107
http://curry.edschool.virginia.edu/commdis/
Program Offerings: **i, iii, v, vii**

## WASHINGTON

EASTERN WASHINGTON UNIVERSITY
Department of Communication Disorders
(509) 359-6622
http://www.csmt.ewu.edu/csmt/cmmd/
    index.html
Program Offerings: **i, iii, v**

UNIVERSITY OF WASHINGTON
Department of Speech & Hearing Sciences
(206) 543-7974
http://depts.washington.edu/sphsc/
Program Offerings: **i, iii, iv, v, vi, vii**

WASHINGTON STATE UNIVERSITY
Department of Speech & Hearing Sciences
(509) 335-4526
http://www.libarts.wsu.edu/speechhearing/
Program Offerings: **i, iii, iv, v, vi, x**

WESTERN WASHINGTON UNIVERSITY
Communication Sciences and Disorders
(360) 650-3855
http://www.ac.wwu.edu/~csd/
Program Offerings: **i, iii, iv, v**

MARSHALL UNIVERSITY
Department of Communication Disorders
(304) 696-3640
http://www.marshall.edu/commdis/
Program Offerings: **i, iii, v**

## WEST VIRGINIA

WEST VIRGINIA UNIVERSITY
Department of Speech Pathology & Audiology
(304) 293-4241
http://www.wvu.edu/~speechpa/
Program Offerings: **i, iii, iv, v**

## WISCONSIN

MARQUETTE UNIVERSITY
Department of Speech-Language Pathology
    & Audiology

(414) 288-3428
http://www.marquette.edu/chs/sppa/
Program Offerings: **i, iii, v, x**

UNIVERSITY OF WISCONSIN, EAU CLAIRE
Department of Communication Disorders
(715) 836-4186
http://www.uwec.edu/Cdis/
Program Offerings: **i, iii, v**

UNIVERSITY OF WISCONSIN, MADISON
Department of Communicative Disorders
(608) 262-3951
http://www.comdis.wisc.edu/
Program Offerings: **i, iii, iv, v, vi, vii**

UNIVERSITY OF WISCONSIN, MILWAUKEE
Department of Communication Sciences and
    Disorders
(414) 229-4263
http://cfprod.imt.uwm.edu/chs/
Program Offerings: **i, iii, v, vii**

UNIVERSITY OF WISCONSIN, RIVER FALLS
Department of Communicative Disorders
(715) 425-3830
http://www.uwrf.edu/comm-dis/
Program Offerings: **i, iii, v**

UNIVERSITY OF WISCONSIN, STEVENS
    POINT
School of Communicative Disorders
(715) 346-2328
http://www.uwsp.edu/commd/
Program Offerings: **i, iii, iv, v**

UNIVERSITY OF WISCONSIN, WHITEWATER
Center for Communicative Disorders
(262) 472-5202
http://academics.uww.edu/commdis/
Program Offerings: **i, iii, v**

## WYOMING

UNIVERSITY OF WYOMING
Division of Communication Disorders
(307) 766-5710
http://uwadmnweb.uwyo.edu/Comdis/
Program Offerings: **i, iii, iv, v, vi, vii**

# APPENDIX C

## Suggested Readings

Bellis, T. J. (2002). *When the brain can't hear: Unraveling the mystery of auditory processing disorder.* New York: Pocket Books.

Brown, C. (1954). *My left foot.* London: Secker & Warburg.

Gannon, J. R. (1981). *Deaf heritage: A narrative history of deaf America.* Silver Spring, MD: National Association of the Deaf.

Keller, H. (1990). *The story of my life.* New York: Bantam.

Keyes, D. (1966). *Flowers for Algernon.* London: Cassell.

Lane, H., Hoffmeister, R., Bahan, B., & Bahan, B. (1996). *A journey into the deaf world.* San Diego, CA: Dawnsign Press.

Murray, F. P., & Goodwillie, S. (1980). *A stutterer's story.* Danville, IL: Interstate Printers & Publishers.

Romoff, A. (2000). *Hear again: Back to life with a cochlear implant.* New York: League for the Hard of Hearing.

Schultz, J.T. (2000). *My walkabout.* Oceanside, CA: Academic Communication Associates.

Sienkiewicz-Mercer, R. (1989). *I raise my eyes to say yes.* Boston: Houghton Mifflin.

Sparks, N. (2000). *The rescue.* New York: Warner Books.

St. Louis, K. O. (2001). *Living with stuttering: Stories, basics, resources, and hope.* Morgantown, WV: Populore.

Thompson, C. E. (1999). *Raising a handicapped child: A helpful guide for parents of the physically disabled.* Oxford, England: Oxford University Press.

Van Cleve, J., & Crouch, B. (1989). *A place of their own: Creating the Deaf community in America.* Washington, DC: Gallaudet University Press.

# Clinical Genres in Writing for the Clinical Practicum

| Clinical Documentation | Description | Function |
|---|---|---|
| **Objectives** (Benchmarks, Goals, Functional Outcomes) | Specific goals around which treatment is based. The traditional form requires that the objectives be measurable and objective. Standard components are: <br> • *Skill:* the target behavior/competency. <br> • *Conditions:* the situations and degree of support anticipated for the individual to successfully demonstrate the skill. <br> • *Criteria:* a quantitative or qualitative means of tracking progress. The anticipated degree of success and independence the individual will achieve. | • Identify areas of priority to be addressed in treatment. <br> • Provide a vision for what is to be accomplished to improve the individual's communication skills. <br> • Afford a means for measuring growth. |
| **Daily Notes** (Lesson Plans, SOAP Notes, Progress Notes, Consultation Note, Assessment/ Treatment Checklists) | A record of each treatment session. May take a variety of forms depending on the setting. These are very brief notations that basically document that the service was provided, along with some information on progress with respect to treatment goals. | • Verifies that an individual received treatment. <br> • Date is always required. <br> • Time of day and length of session may also be mandated. <br> • Tracks progress. <br> • May include plans for the next session. |
| **Annual Treatment Plans** (Individualized Family Service Plan [IFSP] for early intervention, Individualized Educational Plan [IEP] for school age, Individualized Service Plan [ISP] for adults) | A collaborative document that outlines an array of services and supports. Written for and by families with input from any relevant disciplines. Includes starting points and end points for intervention on a yearly basis. | • Ensures that children and adults with disabilities will receive appropriate support services under guidelines established by federal law. <br> • A type of contract that outlines information on an individual's needs and how they will be addressed. |
| **Insurance Forms** | Forms submitted to third-party payers. Generally include clients' personal data, as well as numerical codes for type of problem and service, along with dates and times. | • Allows for reimbursement for services. |
| **Daily Records** (Attendence Logs, Clinical Hours, Schedules) | These records document the amount of time the clinician and client spend in therapy, and track appointments. | • Verifies that services were provided and/or that clinical hours were earned. <br> • Schedules allow for time management and reminders of appointments. |

*(continues)*

*(continued)*

| Clinical Reports | Description | Function |
|---|---|---|
| **Diagnostic Report** | When a client first comes to the clinic, his or her speech, language, and hearing are evaluated, and this document reports the evaluations. It could be written at any point in the semester, and is often cowritten, as students often work in a team to conduct testing. The parts of the report include *background information* (about the client's medical and speech therapy history), *types of tests conducted, description of each test, results from each test, summary of the results, clinical impressions* (the clinician's observations during testing), and *recommendations for therapy* based on the results. | ● Confirms or rules out communication disorders, differences, or delays, to determine the severity of the problem and to make recommendations for services. <br> ● provides baseline data for planning treatment. |
| **Treatment Plan** | Written during the first few weeks of the semester, this document contains the following sections: *background information* (about the client's medical and speech therapy history), *goals* (for speech therapy), *rationales* (reasons for choosing the goals), *level of performance at beginning of semester* (to serve as a baseline), *objectives* (a breakdown of each goal), *program steps* (a breakdown of the steps that will be taken to achieve an objective), and approaches/procedures (a description of the treatment techniques the clinician will use). | ● Outlines the direction therapy will take that semester. <br> ● Is reviewed and signed by the student clinician, clinical supervisor, and client or client's guardian. |
| **Progress Report** | Written at the end of the semester, this document contains all the sections that the treatment plan used, but now includes results of each objective, summary of all the results, clinical impressions (observations made by the clinician and others who communicate regularly with the client), and recommendations (whether or not therapy should continue, what to focus on during the next semester, whether more evaluation should take place, whether the client should get support from other professionals, such as audiologists or occupational therapists). | ● Allows the clinician to review the progress with the client. <br> ● Provides a starting point for the next clinician. <br> ● Communicates results to multiple audiences |

## Clinical Report Revision Guide

**Name:** _____   **Date:** _____

Use this checklist as a guide for reviewing and editing your reports. Submit a copy of this guide with the first drafts of reports that you submit to the Writing Fellow and your supervisors.

|  | Yes | No | Comments |
|---|---|---|---|
| As I was composing this report, adjusted my writing with the intended audiences in mind by . . . |  |  |  |
| I used specialized/technical language when appropriate. When I did so, I provided brief definitions, examples, or context. |  |  |  |
| I reviewed this report to make sure that it is well-organized and chronologically accurate. |  |  |  |
| I eliminated unnecessary words and extraneous information. |  |  |  |
| I used simple sentences when appropriate. |  |  |  |
| I avoided excessive use of passive voice. |  |  |  |
| I used first-person pronouns (I, we) only when appropriate. |  |  |  |

*(continues)*

*(continued)*

| | Yes | No | Comments |
|---|---|---|---|
| I proofread this report for spelling, grammar, and punctuation. | | | |
| I included phonetic symbols if needed. | | | |
| I shared this report with another person for feedback (while maintaining confidentiality) and discovered . . . | | | |
| I read this report aloud and noticed . . . | | | |
| ***For Progress Reports*** | **Yes** | **No** | **Comments** |
| I have adjusted identifying information and background sections to reflect any changes since the treatment plan by . . . | | | |
| I have adjusted the verb tense of each section as needed. | | | |

Which part of the report was easiest to write? Why?

_____

_____

Which part of the report was the most challenging to write? Why?

_____

_____

_____

If I had more time, I would change/revise . . .

_____

_____

_____

## Key Acronyms and Phrases Used in CSD

| | | | |
|---|---|---|---|
| AAA | American Academy of Audiology | EC | Executive Council |
| AAS | American Auditory Society | FAFSA | Free Application for Federal |
| ABD | All But Dissertation | | Student Aid |
| ACPCA | American Cleft Palate-Craniofacial | GPA | Grade point average |
| | Association | GSF | Graduate School Fair |
| ADA | Americans with Disabilities Act | GUR | General University Requirement |
| AIC | Asian Indian Caucus | IDEA | Individuals with Disabilities |
| ANCDS | Academy of Neurological | | Education Act |
| | Communication Disorders and | IEP | Individual Education Plan |
| | Sciences | IRB | Institutional Review Board |
| APA | American Psychological | LC | Legislative Council |
| | Association | LSA | Linguistic Society of America |
| API | Asian Pacific Islander | MA | Master's of Arts |
| ARO | Association for Research in | MS | Master's of Science |
| | Otolaryngology | NAFDA | National Association of Future |
| ASA | Acoustical Society of America | | Doctors of Audiology |
| ASHA | American Speech-Language- | NAPP | National Association of |
| | Hearing Association | | Pre-Professional Programs |
| ASHF | American Speech-Language- | NBASLH | National Black Association for |
| | Hearing Foundation | | Speech-Language and Hearing |
| ASL | American Sign Language | NBGSA | National Black Graduate Student |
| Au.D. | Doctorate of Audiology | | Association, Inc. |
| BA | Bachelor's of Arts | NESPA | National Examination in Speech- |
| BHS | Bachelor's of Health Sciences | | Language Pathology and |
| BHSM | Better Hearing and Speech Month | | Audiology |
| BS | Bachelor's of Sciences | NIH | National Institutes of Health |
| CAOHC | Council for Accreditation in | NSF | National Science Foundation |
| | Occupational Hearing | NSSLHA | National Student Speech |
| | Conservation | | Language Hearing Association |
| CAPCSD | Council for Academic Programs in | OT | Occupational therapist or |
| | Communication Sciences and | | occupational therapy |
| | Disorders | PAC | Political Action Committee |
| CCC | Certificate of Clinical Competence | PET | Positron emission topography |
| CEU | Continuing education unit | Ph.D. | Doctorate of Philosophy |
| CF | Clinical fellowship | PT | Physical therapist or physical |
| CFP | Call for Papers | | therapy |
| CLD | Culturally and linguistically | Quals | Qualifying examinations |
| | different | RC | Regional Councilor |
| CSD | Communication sciences and | SHS | Speech, language, and hearing |
| | disorders | | scientist |
| CV | Curriculum vitae | SLP | Speech-language pathologist |
| DIVISIONS | Special Interest Divisions | SLP-A | Speech-language-pathology |
| EB | Executive Board | (SLPA) | assistant |

# Index

# NSSLHA New Member Application

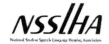

**NSSLHA**
National Student Speech Language Hearing Association

1. Use this application form if you are a new member to NSSLHA. Additional copies can be downloaded from *www.nsslha.org/join*.
2. If your membership in NSSLHA has lapsed or you have not received your renewal notice, renew online at *http://store.asha.org/*
3. Please print information clearly with a ball-point pen.
4. Fax to **(301) 571-0457**; or mail to: **NSSLHA, 10801 Rockville Pike, Rockville, MD 20852;** or call the **ASHA Action Center at 800-498-2071.**

☐ MISS   ☐ MR.   ☐ MRS.   ☐ MS.

FIRST NAME                      MIDDLE INITIAL   LAST NAME

AREA CODE   TELEPHONE                           SSN (OPTIONAL)

_____ @ _____
E-MAIL ADDRESS

CURRENT ACADEMIC INSTITUTION (Enter the institution code under "Current Degree Program" below.)

## Mailing Address for Publications and Correspondence (This is my ☐ home ☐ school ☐ work)

STREET ADDRESS

SECOND LINE OF STREET ADDRESS

CITY

STATE          ZIP CODE          (IF KNOWN)

COUNTRY (IF OTHER THAN THE UNITED STATES)

## Current Degree Program

See degree codes and area of study codes below. For institution code, see www.nsslha.org/join.

|  | Degree Designator | Area of Study | Date Expected or Conferred (MM/YY) | Institution Code |
|---|---|---|---|---|
| DOCTORAL |  |  | / |  |
| MASTERS |  |  | / |  |
| BACHELOR |  |  | / |  |
| ASSOCIATE |  |  | / |  |

### Degree Designator

AA   Associate of Arts
AS   Associate of Science
AAS   Associate of Applied Science
BA   Bachelor of Arts
BS   Bachelor of Science
BE   Bachelor of Education
OB   Other Bachelor's Degree
MA   Master of Arts

MS   Master of Science
ME   Master of Education
OM   Other Master's Degree
AuD   Doctor of Audiology
PhD   Doctor of Philosophy
ScD   Doctor of Science
EdD   Doctor of Education
OD   Other Doctorate

### Areas of Study

AUD   Audiology
OTH   Other
SCI   Speech-Language-Hearing Science
SLA   Speech-Language Pathology Assistant
SLP   Speech-Language Pathology
SPA   Speech-Language Pathology and Audiology

**[Continued on other side]**

## Special Interest Divisions

☐ I want to join an ASHA Special Interest Division(s):

Affiliation in each Special Interest Division is $10 for members of national NSSLHA.
**Include these fees with application.** To learn more about the Special Interest Divisions, please visit **http://www.asha.org**.

☐ Division 1   Learning and Education
☐ Division 2   Neurophysiology and Neurogenic Speech and Language Disorders
☐ Division 3   Voice and Voice Disorders
☐ Division 4   Fluency and Fluency Disorders
☐ Division 5   Speech Science and Orofacial Disorders
☐ Division 6   Hearing and Hearing Disorders: Research and Diagnostics
☐ Division 7   Aural Rehabilitation and Its Instrumentation
☐ Division 8   Hearing Conservation and Occupational Audiology

☐ Division 9   Hearing and Hearing Disorders in Childhood
☐ Division 10   Issues in Higher Education
☐ Division 11   Administration and Supervision
☐ Division 12   Augmentative and Alternative Communication
☐ Division 13   Swallowing and Swallowing Disorders (Dysphagia)
☐ Division 14   Communication Disorders and Sciences in Culturally and Linguistically Diverse (CLD) Populations
☐ Division 15   Gerontology
☐ Division 16   School-Based Issues

## ASHA Journal Selection

In addition to the NSSLHA publications and *The ASHA Leader,* I select the following ASHA journal as my member benefit:

☐ *American Journal of Audiology (AJA)*
☐ *American Journal of Speech-Language Pathology (AJSLP)*
☐ *Journal of Speech, Language and Hearing Research (JSLHR)*
☐ *Language, Speech, and Hearing Services in Schools (LSHSS)*

Please allow 2 to 4 weeks to process the membership and journal selections.

---

### Complimentary Subscription Offer for Students

☐ I am not able to join national NSSLHA at this time but I would like to receive a complimentary subscription to **News & Notes** and further information about NSSLHA.

This is a one-time, one-year subscription to **News & Notes**. Please allow 4 to 6 weeks to process your subscription request.

---

### Ethnicity / Race (optional)

NSSLHA follows federal guidelines on ethnic and racial categories. Please describe BOTH your ethnicity and race, selecting from the federal categories given below.

ETHNICITY
Which of the following describes your ethnicity?
☐ Hispanic or Latino
☐ Not Hispanic or Latino

RACE
Which of the following describes your race? Select all that apply.
☐ American Indian or Alaska Native
☐ Asian
☐ Black or African-American
☐ Native Hawaiian or other Pacific Islander
☐ White

---

**Membership Dues.** (Make check payable to **ASHA**. Membership dues are non-refundable.)

Membership dues (January–December)     **$45**

Special Interest Divisions (optional)    _____ x $10 each =   _____

**TOTAL AMOUNT PAID**    _____

## Method of Payment

☐ Check enclosed. (Payment must be made in U.S. Dollars.)

☐ Please charge my:    ☐ Visa    ☐ Mastercard

---

CREDIT CARD NUMBER        EXPIRATION DATE

---

SIGNATURE

You can join NSSLHA at the same time you register for the ASHA Convention at http://www.asha.org.